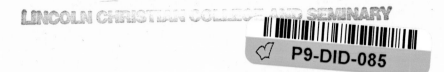

P9-DID-085

Systems of Care for Children's Mental Health

Series Editors:
Beth A. Stroul, M.Ed.
Robert M. Friedman, Ph.D.

What Works in Children's Mental Health Services?

Other Volumes in This Series

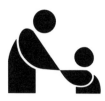

What Works in Children's Mental Health Services?

Uncovering Answers to Critical Questions

by

Krista Kutash, Ph.D.
Deputy Director

and

Vestena Robbins Rivera, M.A.
Research Associate

Research and Training Center for Children's Mental Health
Florida Mental Health Institute
University of South Florida
Tampa

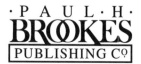

·P A U L·H·
BROOKES
PUBLISHING CO.

Baltimore • London • Toronto • Sydney

Paul H. Brookes Publishing Co.
Post Office Box 10624
Baltimore, Maryland 21285-0624

Typeset by PRO-IMAGE Corporation, York, Pennsylvania.
Manufactured in the United States of America by
The Maple Press Company, York, Pennsylvania.

Library of Congress Cataloging-in-Publication Data
Kutash, Krista.
    What works in children's mental health
services? uncovering answers to critical
questions / by Krista Kutash
and Vestena Robbins Rivera.
      p. cm.—(Systems of care for children's mental health)
    Includes bibliographical references and index.
    ISBN 1-55766-254-1
    1. Child mental health services. 2. Child mental health services—
Research. I. Rivera, Vestena Robbins. II. Series.
RJ499.K88 1996
362.2'083—dc20   96-12812
                                                   CIP

British Library Cataloguing-in-Publication data are available from the
British Library.

Contents

98224

Series Preface

In 1982, Knitzer's seminal study, *Unclaimed Children*, was published by the Children's Defense Fund. At that time, the field of children's mental health was characterized by a lack of federal or state leadership, few community-based services, little collaboration among child-serving systems, negligible parent involvement, and little or no advocacy on behalf of youngsters with emotional disorders. Since that time, substantial gains have been realized in both the conceptualization and the implementation of comprehensive, community-based systems of care for children and adolescents with serious emotional disorders and their families.

A vast amount of information has emanated from the system-building experiences of states and communities and from research and technical assistance efforts. Many of the trends and philosophies emerging in recent years have now become widely accepted as the "state of the art" for conceptualizing and providing services to youngsters with emotional disorders and their families. There is now broad agreement surrounding the need to create community-based systems of care throughout the United States for children and their families, and the development of these systems has become a national goal. Such systems of care are based on the premises of providing services in the most normative environments, creating effective interagency relationships among the key child-serving systems, involving families in all phases of the planning and delivery of services, and creating service systems that are designed to respond to the needs of culturally diverse populations.

A major need is to incorporate these concepts and trends into the published literature. This need stems from the critical shortage of staff who are appropriately trained to serve youngsters in community-based systems of care, with new philosophies and new service delivery approaches. Of utmost importance is the need to provide state-of-the-art information to institutions of higher education for use in the preservice education of professionals across disciplines, including the social work, counseling, psychology, and psychiatry fields. Similarly, there is an equally vital need for resources for the in-service training of staff in mental health, child welfare, education, health, and juvenile justice agencies to assist the staff in working more effectively with youngsters with emotional disorders and their families.

This book series, *Systems of Care for Children's Mental Health*, is designed to fulfill these needs by addressing current trends in children's mental health service delivery. The series has several broad goals:

• To increase awareness of the system-of-care concept and philosophy among current and future mental health professionals who will be providing services to children, adolescents, and their families.

• To broaden the mental health field's understanding of treatment and service delivery beyond traditional approaches to include innovative, state-of-the-art approaches.

• To provide practical information that will assist the mental health field to implement and apply the philosophy, services, and approaches embodied in the system-of-care concept.

Each volume in this continuing series addresses a major issue or topic related to the development of systems of care. The books contain information useful to planners, program managers, policy makers, practitioners, parents, teachers, researchers, and others who are interested and involved in improving systems of care for children with emotional disorders and their families. As the series editors, it is our goal for the series to provide an ongoing vehicle and forum for exploring critical aspects of systems of care as they continue to evolve.

REFERENCE

Knitzer, J. (1982). *Unclaimed children: The failure of public responsibility to children and adolescents in need of mental health services.* Washington, DC: Children's Defense Fund.

Editorial Advisory Board

Foreword

This thorough review of state-of-the-art mental health services for children reflects a burgeoning set of clinical interventions with up-to-date evaluation and research. The usefulness of these services to children and families was carefully assessed. While lagging behind the research base on adult mental health services, the growth of the child mental health services literature since 1990 is impressive, as is the development of new ideas, the presence of investigators prepared to study them, and governmental and foundation support making both possible. In a nascent field, differentiating between what works and what does not work is a complex task that risks reaching premature conclusions. The authors have avoided this problem by describing the studies and their findings, while reserving judgment about these interventions until they can be more thoroughly investigated.

What Works in Children's Mental Health Services? creates an implicit case not just for more, or more sophisticated, research, but for careful consideration of an appropriate research strategy. The classic paradigm, utilized in child psychotherapy research, of moving from laboratory-based clinical trials of efficacy to studies of effectiveness in naturalistic settings, may be neither feasible nor desirable for community-based interventions where narrow exclusion criteria and manualized treatments could be so artificial as to render the findings lacking in external validity. For innovative interventions, such as case management and wraparound services, operationalizing the concepts underlying these interventions and developing clinical protocols and measures of fidelity are prerequisites to further research.

Further issues of research design will benefit from guidance from the field. These include the readiness of clinical interventions for feasibility and uncontrolled studies in contrast to more demanding controlled studies. For controlled studies, subsequent decisions involve choices between randomized and matched designs. Selection of the most appropriate comparison conditions in such studies (i.e., whether to utilize standard care or more promising comparison interventions) will have implications for the likelihood of differential outcomes.

The child services research base presented is relevant to policy deliberations. The limited evidence about the effectiveness of the most expensive institutional forms of care—hospitals and residential treatment centers—may further fuel the rationing of such services under managed care and possible Medicaid block grants. Despite the historical availability of such services, questions remain about whether the necessary research has been conducted to truly evaluate their usefulness. It is very possible, however, that research demonstrating the effectiveness of alternatives to institutional care (e.g., intensive home-based services, therapeutic foster care) may quickly eclipse the need for research on traditional institutional services. The widespread adoption and endorsement of interventions, such as case management and family preservation, by policy makers with limited evidence of an impact on client outcomes could result in requests from policy makers for further evidence—particularly as information about the amount of fiscal resources allocated to them becomes more available. Furthermore, increased recognition of the usefulness of more targeted interventions (e.g., family education, skills training, behavioral approaches) may be understood and acted upon.

Examination of the relationship between the effectiveness of specific interventions and service system characteristics was strongly endorsed. Under impending policies for financing mental health services, if child mental health resources shift from institutional settings to community-based systems of care (without decreasing total dollars) the opportunities to improve our understanding of intervention/system level relationships will increase. Although not sufficient to produce positive clinical outcomes, system level characteristics, such as availability and coordination of services, cultural sensitivity, and family involvement, are essential to the receipt of appropriate care for youth and families in need. Service systems studies will not, however, solve the problem of lack of outcomes for specific interventions. While system level characteristics clearly influence access to services and patterns of service use, and further research on the effectiveness of systems is needed, linking this type of research to client outcomes may be risky unless the clinical interventions are carefully implemented and monitored. Absent the preceding conditions, parallel tracks of research may be more reasonable until the research base for both systems and clinical interventions is more strongly established. To advance our understanding of what works for children and families, it is crucial to concentrate research on the effectiveness of specific interventions (separate and in combination), of which there are multiple promising candidates, and to evaluate whether they also work in the real world of clinical practice. These community-based interventions, lacking the protections offered by the hospital or the office, require multiple high-level skills for which adequate preparation is usually not provided in graduate school or in more clinical settings. Possibly the single exception for combining research on systems and clinical interventions is the case in which the clinical intervention constitutes a system of care (e.g., wraparound services).

In conclusion, this book provides a strong stimulus to researchers for further research. For policy makers, it will assist in decision making; for students, it offers a helpful introduction to innovative child interventions that are not well described in textbooks. *What Works in Children's Mental Health Services?* will move research on the effectiveness of child mental health services forward while providing policy makers, clinical educators, and clinicians with clues about where to invest resources until more definitive answers become available.

Barbara J. Burns, Ph.D.
Duke University Medical Center
Department of Psychiatry and Behavioral Sciences
Durham, North Carolina

Preface

A number of significant changes in the way children and youth with serious emotional disorders and their families are served have occurred since the mid-1980s. One of the major shifts in service delivery has been that toward the building of community-based systems of care. The widely recognized system of care model proposed by Stroul and Friedman (1986, 1994) assumes that, to best meet the needs of children and families, services should be delivered in the least restrictive setting appropriate and should range from residential to nonresidential. The model presents a framework consisting of seven major service dimensions—mental health, social, educational, health, vocational, recreational, and operational —each representing an area of need for children and families. Within each of these service dimensions is an array of service components that serve as building blocks within the system of care. Research has been given a prominent role in the continuing development and revision of the system of care model. The model is "designed to be a guide, based on the best available empirical data and clinical experience to date. It is offered as a starting point . . . as a baseline from which changes can be made as additional research, experience and innovation dictate" (Stroul & Friedman, 1986, p. 29). More recently, Burns (1994) again suggested that evaluation and research on the components within a system of care are essential building blocks within the system of care philosophy.

Given this role of research in the refinement and evolution of a system of care, the next logical step is to determine what the research "says." While research and evaluation play a vital part in service development, often the results are not easily obtainable and thus may not affect service development. Too often, research and evaluation results are not contained within a single, easily accessible resource, but are found within multiple articles, journals, books, reports, and monographs or communicated through presentations at conferences and workshops. Even if an interested party has the time and energy to invest in gathering the written documents, this information must then be synthesized and integrated. If findings are not integrated, some research efforts may be overlooked. This may lead to a number of projects attempting to answer the same questions, rather than building a research base that helps to improve service delivery for children and families.

The current effort was undertaken because we believe that research in the children's mental health services field will contribute to refinements and improvements in the service delivery system. In addition, we believe that many of the current mechanisms used to disseminate research and evaluation results do not reach the targeted audiences for which they may have the greatest impact. Many of the service components discussed within this book are new and have been developed and researched by people in communities, rather than university-based settings as is commonly the case. Thus, the purpose of this book is to serve as a clear, concise summary of the research and evaluation efforts on the service components within a system of care for children and youth.

This book reviews literature on six mental health service components as well as two operational service components in a system of care for children. These components include residential, outpatient (psychotherapy), day treatment, family preservation, therapeutic foster care, crisis/emergency, case management/service coordination, and family support. Given that many of the service components examined within the book are relatively new, we felt it important that each chapter should include a definition of the component in each chapter along with the summary of outcome and empirically based efficacy studies, conclusions, and future research needs. It is our hope that the inclusion of such definitions will help clarify and disseminate their use.

This book is a revision of an earlier monograph titled "Components of a System of Care: What Does the Research Say?" (Rivera & Kutash, 1994). The previous product and this current effort are both partially supported by a grant from the Center for Mental Health Services and the National Institute on Disability and Rehabilitation Research (HB 133B40023). The earlier monograph was distributed to researchers, policy makers, practitioners, advocates, and parents. That monograph, either in part or in total, has been included as text material in a number of academic classes within various disciplines, including psychology, special education, social work, and public health at several universities. Overall, the response to this summary of the research results has been positive and supports the role of research in understanding the service system for children with serious emotional disorders and their families.

It is our hope that the dissemination of this information to parents, service providers, and policy makers may, in some way, assist in the effort to improve mental health services for children and youth with serious emotional disorders and their families.

REFERENCE

Rivera, V.R., & Kutash, K. (1994). *Components of a system of care: What does the research say?* Tampa: University of South Florida, Florida Mental Health Institute, Research and Training Center for Children's Mental Health.

Acknowledgments

At various stages, many individuals participated in and contributed to the development of this product. First, the authors wish to recognize the special contribution of Robert Friedman for his leadership, insight, and guidance during the development of the initial monograph, from which this book was an outgrowth, and his continued support throughout the production of the book.

Each chapter of the initial monograph was reviewed by experts in their respective area of children's mental health. It is to these 15 people that we owe our gratitude for their contribution of time and valuable insight into this endeavor. We wish to express our thanks to the following reviewers: Karen Blase, Barbara J. Burns, John Curry, Lucille Eber, Mary Evans, Glenda Fine, Steven Forness, Pam Meadowcroft, Janice Moore, Carole Pastore, Steven Pfieffer, Barbara Thomlison, John Weisz, Kathleen Wells, and Susan Yelton.

The dedication and assistance of the staff of the Research and Training Center for Children's Mental Health at the Florida Mental Health Institute, University of South Florida, is greatly appreciated. Our gratitude is extended to Kimberly Hall, Ronda Hathaway, and Allison Metcalf, who graciously edited earlier drafts of this product. Furthermore, we gratefully recognize the assistance of Al Duchnowski, Cindy Liberton, George Shuttleworth, Lucy Doyle, Jeff Anderson, and Lynda Bryan.

We also wish to thank Larry Schonfeld for his suggestion to expand the earlier monograph to a book as well as his recommendations and comments throughout this process. A tremendous debt of gratitude is extended to our family and friends for their continuous encouragement and support throughout the duration of this project.

In addition, we want to acknowledge the contribution of Barbara J. Burns, who graciously agreed to write the foreword to this book, as well as that of Lynn Weber, Jennifer Lazaro, and the staff at Paul H. Brookes Publishing Co. who patiently guided us through each phase of the publication process. Finally, we wish to applaud the researchers, both those acknowledged in this book and the many others, who continually strive to increase research efforts and disseminate results that will improve services and enhance the lives of children with serious emotional disorders and their families.

Krista Kutash
Vestena Robbins Rivera

*This book is dedicated
to our parents and grandparents,
who instilled in us the value
of asking questions and being guided by fact.*

*K.K.
V.R.R.*

What Works in
Children's Mental
Health Services?

Introduction

Since the mid-1980s, a number of changes have occurred in the way we serve children with serious emotional disorders and their families. This period of transition has been described as involving a shift in both conceptualization and practice (Duchnowski & Kutash, 1993; Knitzer, 1993). Knitzer (1993) described four shifts related to the areas of family participation, intensity of services, cultural sensitivity, and the development of community-based systems of care. The first shift involves a new conceptualization of the role of the family. Traditionally, families have been viewed as the "cause" of the problems experienced by their children. However, since the mid-1980s, active efforts have been made to eliminate this stereotype, and attempts have begun to have families participate more fully in the treatment planning process for their children. A second shift involves a transformation in the conceptualization of service intensity. Previously, it was thought that intensive services could be provided only by placing children in secure residential settings away from their parents and community. Currently, the development of new services, such as family preservation and individualized, wraparound services, has allowed children to receive intensive services in a natural setting. The third shift pertains to the development of culturally competent service delivery systems. The development of culturally sensitive services requires an acknowledgment of cultural differences as well as the formulation of services that meet the needs of families of color. The fourth shift is concerned with the development and implementation of community-based systems of care, described more fully in the following section.

SYSTEMS OF CARE

A system of care has been defined as

> a comprehensive spectrum of mental health and other necessary services which are organized into a coordinated network to meet the multiple and changing needs of children and adolescents with severe emotional disturbances and their families. (Stroul & Friedman, 1986, p. xx)

The system of care model proposed by Stroul and Friedman (1986) is based on the belief that services are to be provided in the least restrictive setting that is appropriate to the needs of the child and family. A comprehensive and coordinated array of services ranging from residential to nonresidential settings must be in place to successfully meet the individual needs of the child and family. The model presents a framework comprising eight major dimensions of service, each representing an area of need for children and families (see Table 1).

Within each of the service dimensions is an array of service components that serve as building blocks within the system of care. For example, the mental health dimension consists of both nonresidential (e.g., outpatient services, day treatment) and residential (e.g., therapeutic foster care, inpatient hospitalization) services. A listing of the array of mental health services within a system of care is presented in

---

Table 1. Components within a system of care

- Mental health services
- Social services
- Educational services
- Health services
- Substance abuse services
- Vocational services
- Recreational services
- Operational services

From Stroul, B.A., & Friedman, R.M. (1986). *A system of care for children and youth with severe emotional disturbances* (rev. ed., p. xxix). Washington, DC: Georgetown University Child Development Center, National Technical Assistance Center for Children's Mental Health; reprinted with permission.

Table 2. Mental health services within the components of the system of care

Nonresidential services	Residential services
Prevention	Therapeutic foster care
Early identification and intervention	Therapeutic group care
Assessment	Therapeutic camp services
Outpatient treatment	Independent living services
Home-based services	Residential treatment services
Day treatment	Crisis residential services
Emergency services	Inpatient hospitalization

From Stroul, B.A., & Friedman, R.M. (1986). *A system of care for children and youth with severe emotional disturbances* (rev. ed., p. xxix). Washington, DC: Georgetown University Child Development Center, National Technical Assistance Center for Children's Mental Health; reprinted with permission.

Table 2. Operational services differ somewhat from the other dimensions in that they include a range of support services that tend to cut across the boundaries between different types of services. They are called operational services because of their importance to the overall effective operation of the system. Examples of operational services include case management, family support and self-help groups, advocacy, legal services, transportation, and juvenile justice services. In this book, mental health and operational services are highlighted because of their critical importance for children with emotional and behavioral disorders and their families.

Although there has been considerable discussion of the individual service components within a system of care, it is important to acknowledge that these components are part of an overall system. The boundaries between the various dimensions and components are not always clear and frequently overlap. For example, the difference between intensive family preservation services and home-based crisis and emergency services are not always discerned. As Stroul and Friedman (1986) point out,

> only when the services are enmeshed in a coherent, well-coordinated system, will the needs of youngsters with severe emotional disturbances and their families be met in an appropriate and effective manner. (p. xxviii)

Furthermore, because all services are interrelated, the effectiveness of any one component is related to the availability and effectiveness of all other components. For example, day treatment services may be more effective if crisis or residential services are available within the system of care. Similarly, although each mental health service component is discussed and described in a separate chapter in this book, this approach is not meant to diminish the interrelatedness of the services and the combined effectiveness of these services within the overall system of care.

STUDY DESIGNS

It is noteworthy that Stroul and Friedman (1986) have given research an important role in the development of their system of care model. This proposed model is

> designed to be a guide, based on the best available empirical data and clinical experience to date. It is offered as a starting point . . . as a baseline from which changes can be made as additional research, experience and innovation dictate. (p. 29)

More recently, Burns (1994) again suggested that evaluation and research on the components within a system of care are essential building blocks within the system of care philosophy.

In 1990, Burns and Friedman described two levels at which the effectiveness of a system of care for children and adolescents can be investigated. The first level of research entails the more traditional program evaluation strategies of examining and describing the feasibility, acceptability, and general usefulness of an intervention. Models, challenges, and designs for this level of research have been published and disseminated (see Bickman, 1992; Kutash, Duchnowski, Johnson, & Rugs, 1992; Stroul, 1993). The second level of research used to examine the efficacy of a program requires a controlled experiment in a natural setting. Studies conducted under controlled conditions, by employing either a comparison group or random assignment to different types of treatment, are used to support the belief that the outcomes under investigation resulted from the program and not from an irrelevant cause (i.e., a test of internal validity).

Bickman (1992) points out four threats to internal validity: maturation (effects may be a result of the increasing age of the children), selection (effects may be a result of how subjects were selected); history (effects may be a result of an array of changes, such as changes in the overall service environment while a study is being conducted that may have produced the desired effects); and regression artifacts (changes in subjects result from a natural drift in scores, especially extreme scores, to the mean or average scores). Although studies that are conducted under controlled conditions help to eliminate threats to internal validity, this type of study is often seen as a final stage in the development of a program. In a multitiered model of evaluation, Jacobs (1988) suggested that programs developed within an applied setting should initially examine and establish short-term objectives (e.g., changes over time for program participants) and move toward a program impact phase in which control group or comparison group data can be collected.

Because many of the components within the system of care model are still being developed, the present review provides an overview of the available literature that used either single group or pretreatment/posttreatment designs or studies that were conducted under controlled conditions.

TIME FRAME FOR STUDIES REVIEWED

Burns and Friedman (1990) conducted a review of the research base for child mental health services and concluded that, although there had been an expansion in research that examined children's mental health services, a considerable degree of additional research was needed. One part of the research agenda focused on the examination of the effectiveness of the components within a system of care. The purpose of this book was to add to the literature review conducted by Burns and Friedman (1990) by describing the research published since that time. There are some exceptions, in that articles and reports that are summaries of reviews and meta-analyses were included, and these reviews may reflect studies conducted prior to 1990. These descriptions are intended to add to the knowledge base on the system of care approach, stimulate additional research in this area, and serve as a guide and source of information to communities for building systems of care.

A review of the available research literature on six mental health service components and two operational services within a system of care for children was conducted and synthesized. These mental health service components included the following: outpatient services (psychotherapy), day treatment, home-based services, therapeutic foster care, crisis and emergency services, and residential services. Two operational services components were also reviewed: family support services and case management/service coordination. The review of each component is presented in a manner that may appear to indicate a progression from least restrictive to most restrictive treatment environment; however, within the system of care framework, movement from each component is individualized, and each child and family may move independently from one component to another.

Each review consists of definitions of the components, summaries of outcome and empirically based effectiveness studies, and cost data. Because of the constant pressure within the public sector to examine not only the outcomes of service delivery but also the cost of services, studies were sought that aimed primarily at examining the cost-effectiveness and cost–benefit of each component. Cost-effectiveness and cost–benefit studies, which seek to simultaneously consider outcomes (effectiveness and benefits) and the cost of programs, are just beginning to be conducted within the children's mental health services field. However, perhaps as a natural precursor to this type of analysis, many programs have begun to capture the cost of providing services. Some authors have compared the cost of a particular service type with projected amounts of other services. For example, cost savings associated with the prevention or avoidance of residential treatment was used in many service descriptions. When this approach was used, this type of analysis was labeled as cost comparisons and cost savings, because these analyses do not meet the criteria of carefully controlled cost-effectiveness studies. For a more in-depth discussion of cost-effectiveness and cost–benefit analysis, the reader is referred to Davis and Frank (1992).

METHOD

The sources searched for this review included PsycLIT, ERIC, and Sociofile databases; published and unpublished monographs; in press articles; and the conference proceedings of the Annual Research Conference on Children's Mental Health sponsored by the Research and Training Center for Children's Mental Health, Florida Mental Health Institute, University of South Florida, in Tampa. These sources led to the review of over 30 journals and numerous monographs and reports from around the country. Additionally, an earlier version of each chapter was reviewed by experts in their respective area of children's mental health (e.g., case management, day treatment). These experts also provided a wealth of additional materials to be considered for inclusion in the review.

The dissemination of research results to parents, service providers, and policy makers in the field of children's mental health is an important part of research that is often overlooked. It is our hope that this review of the literature on the effectiveness of the mental health components and operational services in a system of care may stimulate and guide future research endeavors that will ultimately lead to improved services for children with serious emotional disorders and their families.

REFERENCES

Bickman, L. (1992). Designing outcome evaluations for children's mental health services: Improving internal validity. In L. Bickman & D. Rog (Eds.), *Evaluating mental health services for children* (pp. 57–68). San Francisco: Jossey-Bass.

Burns, B.J. (1994). The challenges of child mental health services research. *Journal of Emotional and Behavioral Disorders* 2(4), 254–259.

Burns, B.J., & Friedman, R.M. (1990). Examining the research base for children's mental health services and policy. *Journal of Mental Health Administration, 17*(1), 87–98.

Davis, K.E., & Frank, R.G. (1992). Integrating costs and outcomes. In L. Bickman & D.J. Rog (Eds.), *Evaluating mental health services for children* (pp. 69–84). San Francisco: Jossey-Bass.

Duchnowski, A.J., & Kutash, K. (1993, October). *Developing comprehensive systems for troubled youth: Issues in mental health.* Paper presented at Shakertown Symposium II: Developing Comprehensive Systems for Troubled Youth, Shakertown, KY.

Jacobs, F.H. (1988). The five-tiered approach to evaluation: Context and implementation. In H. Weiss & F.H. Jacobs (Eds.), *Evaluating family programs* (pp. 37–71). New York: Aldine De Grutyer.

Knitzer, J. (1993). Children's mental health policy: Challenging the future. *Journal of Emotional and Behavioral Disorders, 1*(1), 8–16.

Kutash, K., Duchnowski, A.J., Johnson, M., & Rugs, D. (1992). Multi-stage evaluation for a community mental health system for children. *Administration and Policy in Mental Health, 20*(4), 311–322.

Stroul, B.A. (1993). *Systems of care for children and adolescents with severe emotional disturbances: What are the results?* Washington, DC: Georgetown University Child Development Center, National Technical Assistance Center for Children's Mental Health.

Stroul, B.A., & Friedman, R.M. (1986). *A system of care for children and youth with severe emotional disturbances* (rev. ed.). Washington, DC: Georgetown University Child Development Center, National Technical Assistance Center for Children's Mental Health.

CHAPTER 1

Outpatient Services

The most commonly utilized mental health service component for children is outpatient therapy. For the purposes of this chapter, the terms *outpatient therapy* and *outpatient services* are used to refer only to psychotherapy, not to forms of therapy that involve the dispensation of medication. Although there is no widely accepted definition, psychotherapy has been defined by Kazdin (1991) as "an intervention designed to decrease distress, psychological symptoms, and maladaptive behavior or to improve adaptive and prosocial functioning" (p. 785). Outpatient therapy is the least restrictive component along the continuum of care and is usually the first and most frequent type of treatment provided to children and families in need of service (Tuma, 1989). Psychotherapy varies with regard to theoretical approach, ranging from psychodynamic to behavioral or cognitive-behavioral to systemic. Recently a combination of the various approaches has been used frequently. Outpatient therapy also occurs in a variety of settings that may include community mental health centers, outpatient psychiatry departments of hospitals, or private offices and is most often provided by psychiatrists, psychologists, social workers, and counselors. Typically, the child and/or family receives therapy in an office on a regular basis (Stroul & Friedman, 1986). Thus, outpatient therapy allows a child to remain in his or her home, school, and community while continuing to receive mental health services (McKelvey, 1988).

Because outpatient services are delivered in a wide variety of settings, it is difficult to obtain an accurate estimate of the number of children receiving such services. In an examination of mental health service use by adolescents in the 1970s and 1980s, Burns (1991) reported 1986 cross-sectional data for 10- to 18-year-olds. The results revealed that the majority (69%) of adolescents who received treatment were served in outpatient settings. Residential treatment centers, inpatient services, and partial hospitalization services were used by a much smaller percentage of adolescents: 8%, 22%, and 3%, respectively. Burns further examined shifts in the use of services over time. In 1975, a total of 228,584 outpatient admissions (68% of the total admissions to mental health services) were reported, compared with 371,307 (69%) in 1986. Thus, an overall growth rate of 62% in the number of admissions to outpatient services was evident from 1975 to 1986.

Along with a variety of social services, psychotherapy is an intervention that is commonly used in the treatment of children and youth with emotional and behavioral problems (Kazdin, 1993). Although outpatient therapy has an extensive efficacy literature, little attention has been given to the effectiveness of this service in the treatment of children and youth with serious emotional disorders (Burns & Friedman, 1989, 1990). The purpose of this chapter is to provide a brief overview of a number of scholarly reviews of studies examining the effectiveness of child and adolescent psychotherapy. For a more detailed and in-depth discussion of the issues related to outpatient care for children, the reader is referred to Weisz and Weiss (1993).

EFFECTIVENESS AND OUTCOME RESEARCH

Review by Eysenck

The earliest review of the effectiveness of psychotherapy was conducted in 1952 by Eysenck. Based on this review, Eysenck concluded that the use of psychotherapy in the treatment of adults resulted in improvements no greater than those that occurred in the absence of treatment. Although a limited number of studies involving children were included, this initial review led to further investigations of the effectiveness of psychotherapy for children and adolescents (Kazdin, 1991).

Review by Barrnett, Docherty, and Frommelt

In a review of child psychotherapy research conducted since 1963, Barrnett, Docherty, and Frommelt (1991) presented a summary of four reviews. In the earliest review, Levitt noted that the results did not lend support to the use of psychotherapy in the treatment of children. A later review conducted by Wright and his colleagues found that successful outcome status was apparent between termination and follow-up and that improvement was positively correlated with the number of therapy sessions attended. In 1980, Tramontana reviewed the adolescent psychotherapy literature for the period 1967–1977. Thirty-three studies of individual, group, and family therapy were included, although only five of the studies were determined to have employed adequate methodologies. Despite this lack of methodologically sound studies, Tramontana concluded that psychotherapy was effective when compared with no treatment. During the same year, Smith and her colleagues examined control studies using meta-analysis.[1] The analysis revealed that those receiving psychotherapy had outcomes significantly better than those in the control condition.

Review by Weisz and Colleagues

Weisz and his colleagues (Weisz, Donenberg, Han, & Kauneckis, 1995; Weisz, Weiss, & Donenberg, 1992) reviewed four meta-analyses examining the effectiveness of psychotherapy with children and youth. The first meta-analysis reviewed was conducted by Casey and Berman and included 75 studies published during the period of 1952–1983. The studies involved children with a wide range of presenting problems and included a variety of theoretical approaches. Results indicated that children who received psychotherapy showed greater improvement following treatment than did 76% of the children who received no treatment.

The second meta-analysis was conducted by Weisz, Weiss, Alicke, and Klotz and involved a total of 105 outcome studies published between the years of 1952 and 1983. Children included in these studies were between the ages of 4

---

[1] Meta-analysis developed by Glass, McGaw, and Smith (1981) is a "set of quantitative procedures that can be used to evaluate multiple studies" (Kazdin, 1991, p. 786). An effect size, the calculated difference between means of a treatment and control group and divided by the standard deviation of the control group, is computed, which then provides a summary statistic that allows examination of the impact of other variables.

and 18 years, and the majority exhibited either an internalizing or an externalizing disorder. Both behavioral and non-behavioral interventions were used, with the majority of interventions involving a behavioral approach. Similar to the findings of Casey and Berman, the results revealed that children receiving psychotherapy functioned better following treatment than did 79% of those in the control group. It was further concluded that behavioral treatments were more effective than nonbehavioral approaches. It should be noted that this conclusion has been questioned by others in the field—for example, Shirk and Russell (1992), who, based on reviews of the nonbehavioral literature, stated that "such comparisons are, at best, premature" due to a lack of methodologically sound research (p. 707). Similarly, in a review of 43 nonbehavioral (traditional verbal and play therapy) child psychotherapy research studies conducted since 1963, Barrnett et al. (1991) concluded that a large number of methodological flaws were apparent that restricted the accuracy of conclusions regarding the efficacy of these nonbehavioral approaches.

The third meta-analysis included in the review was conducted by Kazdin, Bass, Ayers, and Rodgers and involved studies published between 1970 and 1988. Studies utilized a variety of intervention approaches and involved children who exhibited internalizing, externalizing, and learning-academic problems. A total of 105 studies comparing treatment and control groups were analyzed. For studies involving groups with treatment versus no treatment, children who received treatment exhibited greater improvement than did 81% of those in the control group. For those studies comparing treatment and control groups, children who received treatment functioned better than did 78% of those in the active control group.

Finally, preliminary data resulting from a meta-analysis conducted by Weisz, Weiss, Morton, Granger, and Han were reviewed. This comprehensive review incorporated 110 studies published between 1967 and 1991 that involved children ages 2–18 years. The majority of children exhibited either externalizing or internalizing problems, and the majority of studies involved the use of behavioral interventions. Meta-analytic procedures revealed that, after treatment, children receiving psychotherapy functioned better than did 76% of those in the control group.

Review of Specialty Meta-analyses by Weisz and Colleagues

Five specialty meta-analyses, each focusing on different therapeutic approaches, were reviewed by Weisz and his colleagues (Weisz, Donenberg, Han, & Kauneckis, 1995; Weisz et al., 1992). These studies included an examination of the effectiveness of family therapy as conducted by Hazelrigg, Cooper, and Borduin; a review of studies investigating the effectiveness of cognitive-behavioral therapy with 4- to 13-year-olds conducted by Durlak, Fuhrman, and Lampman; a review of outcome studies that examined the effectiveness of self-statement modification (SSM) with children ages 5–16 years conducted by Dush, Hirt, and Schroeder; a review of outcome studies examining the efficacy of cognitive-behavioral methods in the treatment of child impulsivity conducted by Baer and Nietzel; and an exploration of the impact of child psychotherapy on the language proficiency of children conducted by Russell, Greenwald, and Shirk. Each of these studies provided evidence to support the efficacy of psychotherapy.

As can be seen, meta-analyses have provided a *general* conclusion supporting the effectiveness of psychotherapy with children and adolescents. However, Weisz et al. (1992) have stated that such a conclusion may be premature. That is, most studies on psychotherapy appear to have involved children, interventions, and/or treatment conditions not representative of conventional clinic-based practice. Therefore, it is not known whether the findings derived from the studies conducted under "controlled laboratory settings" can be generalized to therapy conducted in clinics. To that end, Weisz and his colleagues (Weisz, Donenberg, et al., 1995; Weisz & Weiss, 1993; Weisz et al., 1992) reviewed the findings of several clinic-based studies that met certain specifications (see Weisz, Donenberg, et al., 1995, for a description of the criteria used to select studies for inclusion in the review).

Review of Clinic-Based
Studies by Weisz and Colleagues

The first study reviewed was conducted by Shepherd, Oppenheim, and Mitchell in 1966 and examined matched pairs of children; that is, children in treatment were matched with children in the general population (n = 50 pairs). At 2 years after initial assessment, in-home clinical interviews revealed improvements for 63% of the clinic cases and 61% of the non-clinic cases. There was no relationship between the number of treatment sessions and subsequent improvement.

A study by Witmer and Keller was reviewed that compared the outcomes for children who received treatment (n = 85) with those for children who received only a diagnostic evaluation (n = 50). The two groups were followed for 6–13 years after contact with a child guidance clinic. Results indicated that 28% of the children who received treatment were rated as *successful* compared with 48% of those who received only a diagnostic evaluation. A greater percentage (30%) of individuals in the evaluation-only group were rated as *improved*, whereas 26% of those in the treatment group received such a rating. Overall, those who received only an evaluation had better long-term outcomes than did those who received treatment.

Weisz and his colleagues reviewed four clinic-based studies conducted by Lehrman, Sirluck, Black, and Glick in 1949; Levitt, Beiser, and Robertson in 1959; Ashcraft in 1971; and Jacob, Magnussen, and Kemler in 1972. These studies were designed to compare children who did and did not receive treatment, all of whom had been admitted to the same facility during the same period of time, but with the control group comprising children who dropped out before receiving treatment. The earliest study found that at the 1-year follow-up, the percentage of cases classified as successful was significantly higher for those who received treatment (n = 196) than for those in the control group (n = 110), and the percentage of cases rated as failures were greater for those in the control group. The second study assessed outcomes on 26 variables approximately 5 years after clinic contact. No significant differences were noted between the treatment group (n = 237) and the control group (n = 93). Furthermore, no differences were found between the control group and those in the treatment group, who received 10 additional therapy sessions. The third study consisted of a 5-year follow-up study of children receiving treatment (n = 40) and those who dropped out before treatment (n = 43). Outcomes were assessed using measures of academic achievement, because these children had been classified as academic underachievers. No differences were noted between the two groups on any outcome measure. The fourth study compared 45 children who received treatment with 42 children who left the program before receiving treatment. Outcome comparisons conducted at 1- and 2-year follow-up periods revealed no significant differences between the groups.

Weisz and Weiss (1989) conducted a more recent study investigating the efficacy of clinic-based treatment by examining the outcome of treated youth and those who left the program before treatment. In this study, youth (n = 93) from nine clinics who completed a 6-month course of therapy were compared with youth (n = 60) who dropped out of treatment following an intake evaluation. Outcomes were assessed at intake, 6 months following intake, and again at 1 year. Outcome measures included the completion of the Child Behavior Checklist (CBCL) by parents, the parents' identification of the three major problems experienced by their child and the severity of these problems, and the completion of the CBCL Teacher Report Form (TRF) for a subsample of the youth. Results revealed no significant differences between the groups on any measure at 6 months or at 1 year after intake.

Two clinic-based studies that utilized random assignment were reviewed by Weisz, Donenberg, et al. (1995). DeFries, Jenkins, and Williams matched pairs of foster care children with serious disorders as measured on a number of demographic and clinical factors. One member of each pair was randomly assigned to receive standard foster care services, and the other group received psychotherapy and enhanced foster care services. After therapy, children were rated as *improved*, *no change*, or *worsened*. No significant differences were noted between the two groups. Furthermore, institutionalization occurred more frequently among those in the treated group as compared with those in the comparison group. A second and more recent study, conducted by Smyrnios and Kirkby, utilized a random-assignment study. A total of 30 clinic-referred children and their parents were placed in either time-unlimited or time-limited (12 sessions) psychodynamic therapy or in a control group that received minimal contact. After termination of therapy and at 4-year follow-up, some outcome measures revealed no significant differences between the treatment and control groups. Some measures indicated more positive outcomes for those in the minimal contact group than for those in the unlimited treatment group.

CONCLUSIONS AND FUTURE RESEARCH NEEDS
In general, most laboratory-based studies examining the effectiveness of psychotherapy for children found an overall positive effect of treatment. However, it has been argued that these laboratory-based studies failed to accurately represent how therapy and treatment are carried out in "real world" clinic-based settings (Kazdin, Bass, Ayers, & Rodgers, 1990; Weisz, 1988; Weisz, Donenberg, et al., 1995). In fact, the effects of outpatient psychotherapy in clinic-based studies analyzed by meta-analysis and reviewed by Weisz and his colleagues may not be as positive as the findings from meta-analyses of laboratory-based studies. A number of tentative explanations for the disparity between psychotherapy outcomes in experimental (laboratory) versus clinical settings have been provided. Generally, three factors were more common in laboratory-based therapy than in therapy conducted in the clinic: 1) the use of behavioral (including cognitive-behavioral) methods; 2) reliance on specific, focused methods rather than eclectic approaches; and 3) provision of structure, through treatment manuals, for example, and monitoring to foster adherence to treatment plans (see Weisz, Donenberg, et al., 1995, for a complete description of these differences).

Because few of the clinic-based studies were conducted in recent years and because these studies represent a small database, most of which are dated, definite conclusions about the effectiveness of clinic-based therapy compared with laboratory-based therapy cannot yet be drawn. Thus, future research must concentrate upon expanding the base of research on clinic-based psychotherapy and identifying those conditions under which the positive effects of psychotherapy can best be achieved. For a discussion and a meta-analysis on this developing issue, see Weisz, Weiss, Han, Granger, and Morton (1995).

Furthermore, a limited number of studies have been conducted to examine the *specific* treatment approaches that result in beneficial effects for *specific* types of problems. Thus, a second area of needed research is to examine those therapeutic approaches that work most effectively with specific populations of children. A concise summarization of the direction that future research must take has been described by Saxe, Cross, and Silverman (1988) in the following manner:

> The important question may not be about the overall effectiveness of child therapy but about the effectiveness of (a) what therapy, (b) under what conditions, (c) for which children, (d) at which developmental level, (e) with which disorder(s), (f) under what environmental conditions, and (g) with which concomitant parental, familial, environmental, or systems interventions. (p. 803)

REFERENCES

Barrnett, R.J., Docherty, J.P., & Frommelt, G.M. (1991). A review of child psychotherapy research since 1963. *Journal of the American Academy of Child and Adolescent Psychiatry, 30*(1), 1–14.

Burns, B.J. (1991). Mental health service use by adolescents in the 1970s and 1980s. *Journal of the American Academy of Child and Adolescent Psychiatry, 30*(1), 144–150.

Burns, B., & Friedman, R. (1989). The research base for child mental health services and policy: How solid is the foundation? In P. Greenbaum, R. Friedman, A. Duchnowski, K. Kutash, & S. Silver (Eds.), *Conference Proceedings on Children's Mental Health Services and Policy: Building a Research Base* (pp. 7–12). Tampa, FL: University of South Florida, Florida Mental Health Institute, Research and Training Center for Children's Mental Health.

Burns, B., & Friedman, R. (1990). Examining the research base for child mental health services and policy. *Journal of Mental Health Administration, 17*(1), 87–98.

Eysenck, H.J. (1952). The effects of psychotherapy: An evaluation. *Journal of Consulting Psychology, 16*, 319–324.

Glass, G.V., McGaw, B., & Smith, M.L. (1981). *Meta-analysis in social research.* Beverly Hills, CA: Sage Publications.

Kazdin, A. (1991). Effectiveness of psychotherapy with children and adolescents. *Journal of Consulting and Clinical Psychology, 59*(6), 785–798.

Kazdin, A. (1993). Psychotherapy for children and adolescents: Current progress and future research directions. *American Psychologist, 48*(6), 644–657.

Kazdin, A.E., Bass, D., Ayers, W.A., & Rodgers, A. (1990). Empirical and clinical focus of child and adolescent psychotherapy research. *Journal of Consulting and Clinical Psychology, 58,* 729–740.

McKelvey, R. (1988). A continuum of mental health care for children and adolescents. *Hospital and Community Psychiatry, 39*(8), 870–873.

Saxe, L., Cross, T., & Silverman, N. (1988). Children's mental health: The gap between what we know and what we do. *American Psychologist, 43*(10), 800–807.

Shirk, S.R., & Russell, R.L. (1992). A reevaluation of estimates of child therapy effectiveness. *Journal of the American Academy of Child and Adolescent Psychiatry, 31*(4), 703–710.

Stroul, B.A., & Friedman, R.M. (1986). *A system of care for children and youth with severe emotional disturbances* (rev. ed.). Washington, DC: Georgetown University Child Development Center, National Technical Assistance Center for Children's Mental Health.

Tuma, J. (1989). Mental health services for children: The state of the art. *American Psychologist, 44*(2), 188–199.

Weisz, J.R. (1988). Assessing outcomes of child mental health services. *Conference proceedings on children's mental health services and policy: Building a research base* (pp. 38–43). Tampa, FL: University of South Florida, Florida Mental Health Institute, Research and Training Center for Children's Mental Health.

Weisz, J.R., Donenberg, G.R., Han, S.S., & Kauneckis, D. (1995). Child and adolescent psychotherapy outcomes in experiments versus clinics: Why the disparity? *Journal of Abnormal Child Psychology, 23*(1), 83–106.

Weisz, J.R., & Weiss, B. (1989). Assessing the effects of clinic-based psychotherapy with children and adolescents. *Journal of Consulting and Clinical Psychology, 57*(6), 741–746.

Weisz, J.R., & Weiss, B. (1993). *Effects of psychotherapy with children and adolescents.* Newbury Park, CA: Sage Publications.

Weisz, J.R., Weiss, B., & Donenberg, G.R. (1992). The lab versus the clinic: Effects of child and adolescent psychotherapy. *American Psychologist, 47*(12), 1578–1585.

Weisz, J.R., Weiss, B., Han, S.S., Granger, D.A., & Morton, T. (1995). Effects of psychotherapy with children and adolescents revisited: A meta-analysis of treatment outcomes studies. *Psychological Bulletin, 117*(3), 450–468.

CHAPTER 2

Day Treatment and Emerging School-Based Models

According to Stroul and Friedman (1986), day treatment services for children and adolescents are the most intensive form of nonresidential services available. Day treatment is broadly conceptualized as any program falling in the middle of the continuum of care—that is, between inpatient and outpatient treatment (Topp, 1991). Due to this rather broad conceptualization, no universally accepted definition exists. The nature of programs defined as day treatment varies widely with regard to setting, population served, intensity, theoretical approach, and treatment components. For example, the settings vary from hospital based to school based, and the populations served range from children with severe emotional disorders to children with developmental delays. Theoretical approaches also vary; some implement a psychoanalytical approach, and others utilize a behavioral approach.

Stroul and Friedman (1986) defined day treatment as "a service that provides an integrated set of educational, counseling, and family interventions that involve a youngster for at least five hours a day" (p. 44). Through the provision of a broad range of services delivered in a coordinated manner, day treatment programs are designed to strengthen individual and family functioning and to prevent more restrictive placement of children (Research and Training Center for Children's Mental Health, 1985–1986). The term *partial hospitalization*, which refers to hospital-based day treatment programs, has been defined as the "use of a psychiatric hospital setting for less than 24-hour-a-day care" with children returning to their home each night (Tuma, 1989, p. 193). At the other end of the continuum of day treatment programs are school-based day programs. Psychoeducational day school programs have been described as "treatment settings for non-mentally retarded children with severe behavior disorders who are unable to function adaptively in the regular school system" (Baenen, Parris Stephens, & Glenwick, 1986, p. 263). Day school programs usually include collaboration between mental health and special education professionals, a multidisciplinary treatment approach, low student-teacher ratios, service provision to families, and the ultimate goal of reintegration into the educational or vocational mainstream.

Although the specific features of day treatment programs vary widely and no universally accepted definition exists, most include the following components (Stroul & Friedman, 1986):

- Special education, generally in small classes and with a strong emphasis on individualized instruction;
- Counseling, which may include individual and group counseling approaches;
- Family services including family counseling, parent training, brief individual counseling with parents, and assistance with specific tangible needs such as transportation, housing or medical arrangements;
- Vocational training, particularly for adolescents;
- Crisis intervention, not only to assist students through difficult situations but to help them improve problem solving skills;
- Skill building with an emphasis on interpersonal and problem solving skills and practical skills of everyday life;
- Behavior modification with a focus on promoting success through the use of positive reinforcement procedures; and
- Recreational, art and music therapy to further aid in the social and emotional development of the youngsters. (p. 50)

Day treatment services are unique in providing children intensive treatment while they remain in their home and community (LeCroy & Ashford, 1992) and in serving the dual purpose of offering an intensive but less restrictive alternative to hospitalization and providing a means of transition for children moving from inpatient to outpatient care (Tuma, 1989). Furthermore, children may receive day treatment services in combination with community-based residential services to increase the impact of both programs (Stroul & Friedman, 1986).

COST COMPARISONS AND COST SAVINGS

As well as being a less restrictive component in a system of care, day treatment is a less expensive alternative in comparison with residential services. The cost of day treatment for an individual child typically ranges from $10,000 to $15,000 per year, with funding generally provided by multiple sources such as education and mental health programs (e.g., departments of education, mental health agencies) (Stroul & Friedman, 1986). The relative cost savings of day treatment is evident when compared with residential treatment. A number of studies examining the potential cost savings of day treatment/partial hospitalization were conducted during the 1970s. These studies consistently demonstrated the cost savings of partial hospitalization when compared with inpatient treatment (see Parker & Knoll, 1990, for a brief review of these studies).

There is a scarcity of studies, however, comparing the cost of day treatment with residential placement for children and youth. Our literature search found only two studies. The earliest study was conducted by Kiser, Ackerman, and Pruitt (1987) and focused on the relative cost difference of treating children in a day treatment program versus inpatient hospitalization. Findings indicated a significant difference in *daily costs*, with day treatment costing significantly less than inpatient treatment; however, analyses revealed a shorter length of stay for those receiving inpatient treatment than for those in day treatment. Thus, *total costs* for day treatment and hospitalization were found not to be significantly different. However, due to the nature of the data collection procedures used in the study, it is likely that the reported lengths of stay for the inpatient group were underestimated and are thus unreliable. Therefore, the authors conservatively concluded that "day treatment is at least as cost effective as hospitalization and may be significantly more cost effective" (Kiser et al., 1987, p. 25).

A more recent study conducted by Grizenko and Papineau (1992) compared the cost of day treatment with that of residential treatment for children with severe behavior problems. In this study, data were gathered through a retrospective chart/record review that examined cost differences for 23 children admitted to a psychiatric facility for residential treatment and for 23 children admitted to the same facility after it was converted to a day treatment program. The two groups were similar across a number of demographic, family, social support, and treatment variables. Two relevant findings emerged: 1) the average length of stay for those in the day treatment program was significantly shorter than for those in the residential program, and 2) the total cost of treatment for children in the day treatment group was significantly less than for the inpatient residential group. Although a number of methodological limitations were inherent in this study, the authors stated that issues previously neglected in the literature were explored, thus paving the way for future research endeavors in this area.

EFFECTIVENESS AND OUTCOME RESEARCH

Single-Outcome Criteria

The rate of reintegration into general school settings following day treatment has been the most frequently used outcome criterion for evaluating the effectiveness of day treatment programs. Two reviews examining the effectiveness of day treatment and day school programs are available (see Baenen et al., 1986; Zimet & Farley, 1985). Overall, these two reviews revealed that 65%–70% of the children in the studies were reintegrated into general school settings following successful discharge from the day treatment programs. In general, 80% of the children and youth improved on clinical measures, whereas 20% were expelled or sent to a more restrictive setting, such as a residential treatment center (Burns & Friedman, 1990).

In another review conducted by Gabel and Finn (1986), the authors stated that conclusive statements regarding the effectiveness of day treatment for children could not be made. However, based on the literature reviewed, it appears that many children benefit from day treatment, although treatment gains are often modest. Academic and behavioral improvements were noted in a number of studies, and the importance of family involvement during treatment was found to be a critical factor in success.

A more recent review of studies evaluating day treatment programs for children has been conducted by Sayegh and Grizenko (1991). In their review of studies that used rate

of reintegration into general school settings as the single outcome criterion, Sayegh and Grizenko concluded that day
treatment decreased the need for residential placement and
thus reduced cost. The authors cautioned that many of the
studies contained in their review consisted of a heterogene-
ous population and that day treatment may not be effective
with all populations.

Gabel, Finn, and Ahmad (1988) conducted a retrospective study to examine the outcome of a group ($N = 52$)
of predominantly African American children served in a
hospital-based day treatment program in an urban area. The
program served only minority children with severe disturbances from chaotic home environments. The program was
mainly psychodynamic, with a focus on individual and
group psychotherapy. Mental health services were provided
by hospital staff, and educational services were delivered by
the local school district. Data were collected retrospectively
from the records of the children's day hospital over a 5-year
period. Using living arrangement at discharge (home or residential) as the single-outcome criterion, the authors found
that upon discharge 56% of the children were recommended
for residential placement and 44% were recommended for
continued placement in the home. Variables found to be significantly related to residential placement after discharge included a history of child abuse, parental substance abuse,
suicidal behavior, and assaultive/destructive behavior. Day
treatment was found to be effective for certain urban minority children with behavioral difficulties, but less effective if
the variables related to abuse and destructive behavior were
present at admission. A small sample size, restricted population, the use of retrospective data collection procedures, and
the lack of a control group raise important questions about
the generalization of these findings to other day treatment
settings.

Multiple-Outcome Criteria
Studies in the 1990s have been more successful in examining the effectiveness of day treatment through the use of
multiple-outcome criteria. These studies included improvements in behavior and academic performance as outcome criteria, in addition to reintegration into general school settings.

Based on their review of studies using multiple-outcome criteria, Sayegh and Grizenko (1991) concluded that, although improvement rates for students receiving day treatment services were generally around 67%, children continued to require long-term special educational services after discharge. The authors further concluded that day treatment

> is particularly beneficial for children and adolescents with any of the following problems: conduct disorders, attention deficit disorders, adjustment disorders, developmental delays and withdrawn but with normal nonverbal intelligence, and severe emotional disturbances. Children referred to day treatment for severe behavior problems often do not improve and tend to drop out of treatment earlier and more often than other children. (p. 251)

More recent studies reviewed by Sayegh and Grizenko (1991) are summarized briefly here as follows, as well as additional studies not included in their review. Sack, Mason, and Collins (1987) conducted a long-term follow-up study of children enrolled in a psychiatric day treatment center that served children with severe emotional disturbances. The program philosophy was basically psychodynamic, psychoeducational, and milieu oriented. Each child received a comprehensive assessment and individual treatment plan. Children attended small classes staffed by one milieu therapist and a classroom teacher who were supervised by a multidisciplinary team of professionals. Parents often served as classroom volunteers and also received outpatient therapy. A retrospective chart/record review was conducted for each child ($N = 79$) as well as a semistructured follow-up interview with a parent, caregiver, or caseworker to obtain information about the child's current adjustment and behavior, family stability, and use of health and mental health services since discharge. Results revealed that children with emotional disorders (e.g., anxiety, depression) fared better at followup than those children with disorders in the broad category of psychotic or behavioral problems. Family stability was associated with success after discharge. The importance of postdischarge follow-up services and parent involvement during treatment also was noted. The lack of a control group and the use of retrospective chart/record review were limitations inherent in this study.

Cohen and her colleagues have conducted a number of prospective outcome studies evaluating the impact of a therapeutic day treatment program for preschoolers with developmental delays and emotional disorders (ages 3–6 years). These studies have several methodological advantages over other studies, including a prospective design, the use of a control group, the use of standardized measures, and the availability of demographic information (see Sayegh & Grizenko, 1991). In the first study conducted by Cohen, Bradley, and Kolers (1987), a group of 55 children from a therapeutic child care program and 45 children from community child care centers were included in the sample. Children attended the therapeutic preschool for half days 5 days a week for 1–2 years. Interventions were designed by a clinical team and carried out by classroom teachers in a playroom setting. Treatment goals were based on the individual needs of each child, but they most often included the establishment of cognitive, language, social, self-help, and language/communication skills; the establishment of limits on disruptive behavior; and assistance to the child to become a more active participant, to verbally express feelings, and to observe cause–effect relationships. Families were expected to observe and participate in playroom activities under the guidance of staff and to maintain frequent contact with a social worker regarding marital and family issues.

To evaluate the effectiveness of the therapeutic preschool program, a battery of objective developmental, behavioral, and clinical measures was administered at three points during the study: initially, 8–9 months later, and at discharge. Results revealed that children with developmental delays and related emotional and behavioral problems made the most gains, especially those children with nonverbal intelligence in the normal range. Significant gains were not observed for those children who presented primarily behavioral and emotional problems, except for some improvements in impulse control. After discharge, 42% of the children were integrated into general school settings; however, the treatment group did not perform at the level of the control group on psychometric tests. Findings further suggested that interventions for children with developmental delays must be prolonged (up to 2 years of continuous treatment) and that the period of time required for observable gains depends on the area of functioning being considered and the child's level of development at preadmission.

Cohen, Kolers, and Bradley (1987) conducted a second study of 53 children (ages 3–6) at the therapeutic preschool program described previously. The purpose of the study was to identify variables related to treatment outcome in the therapeutic preschool. A battery of measures similar to that of the previous study (see Cohen, Bradley, & Kolers, 1987) was administered 1 month after admission and at discharge. A multiple regression analysis was conducted to examine the relationship between outcome and a number of variables, including initial level of functioning, biological and psychosocial risk indices, age at admission, length of treatment, and degree of parental involvement during treatment. Results indicated that outcome is most positive for children who function at a relatively high level of development, whose families are motivated, who are younger at admission, and who receive treatment for longer than 1 year.

Kosturn, Brown, and Brown (1990) conducted a prospective investigation of the effectiveness of a day treatment program for children with emotional disturbances. The day treatment program accommodated children ages 5–12 years and served only those who exhibited behavior problems *both* at home and at school. Most of the children were classified as having oppositional or conduct disorders. The four major components of the program included day treatment classroom activities, parent training, family therapy, and consultation with school personnel. The program stressed the collaboration of parents, school staff, and therapists in the provision of short-term intensive treatment as an alternative to a more restrictive placement setting. The sample for this study consisted of all children ($N = 75$) admitted to the day treatment program between 1980 and 1985. Complete data were obtained on 23% of the original participants. Standardized parent ratings of child behavior as well as direct classroom observation were used to measure treatment effectiveness. Measures were taken prior to treatment, immediately following discharge, and at 3, 6, and 12 months after termination. Results indicated that day treatment was associated with significant positive gains, as revealed by three standardized parent measures of child behavior. At discharge, parents reported a significant increase in appropriate behavior and a significant decrease in inappropriate behavior by their child. Furthermore, parental reports indicated that inappropriate behavior was less severe after treatment. Treatment gains were evident at follow-up, as revealed by two parent measures administered after termination. No significant change in classroom behavior was observed after treatment; however, this finding has been attributed to the fact that behavior was observed only once before and after treatment and that observation periods were of a brief 30-minute duration. The small number of subjects and the lack of a control group were additional limitations of this study.

Orchard and MacLeod (1990) conducted a 2-year retrospective review of a day program that served adolescents ages 12–19 years. Program components included group and individual therapy, recreational activities, and training in life skills and social skills. In addition, each youth was assigned to a staff person who functioned as a case manager and an in-program therapist. Results were obtained through a review of the records/charts of 97 youth who attended the program over a 2-year period. Attendance and adjustment to community living were used to measure the success of the program. From these outcome measures, the day treatment program was determined to be successful in treating this population of troubled youth. The average rate of attendance was 69%; that is, youth attended the day program approximately 3 out of 4 days. Additionally, improvement in adjustment to community living was observed at discharge. Approximately 80% of the youth were attending school or work, thus indicating an improvement in community functioning. Furthermore, at discharge, almost 77% were living with family or in other community settings, such as group homes or independent living environments. The authors noted, however, that these conclusions should be viewed with caution due to the lack of rigorous methodology.

Two additional studies conducted by Grizenko and colleagues examined the effectiveness of a psychodynamically oriented day treatment program for children with behavior problems (Grizenko, Papineau, & Sayegh, 1993; Grizenko & Sayegh, 1990). Children admitted to this day treatment program received services for an average of 7 months. Treatment goals were individually based, but they often included assisting the child in understanding the cause–effect relationship of family functioning and the child's behavior; allowing the child to express his or her feelings verbally as opposed to behaviorally; building the child's socialization skills, peer relationships, self-esteem, and communication skills; and improving academic performance. Program components included special education services, play therapy, social skills group therapy, psychodrama, and group therapy. On a weekly basis, families received family therapy based on a systemic approach. The dispensation of medication was used when deemed necessary.

In the earlier study (Grizenko & Sayegh, 1990), the investigators examined 23 consecutive admissions to the program using a single-group pretest–posttest design. Children and parents were assessed at admission and discharge using standardized instruments to assess behavioral, academic, demographic, personality, and family variables. Discharge scores revealed a significant improvement on all standardized measures for behavior, academics, personality, and family. Although all children showed improvement, parents reported greater improvements in behavior than did teachers or therapists. Significantly lower rates of improvement were observed for children with conduct disorder than for those with attention-deficit/hyperactivity disorder, oppositional defiant disorder, and depression. Only 17% of the children were attending general school at admission, while 87% of the children had been reintegrated into general school settings at discharge. Findings must be viewed with caution due to a number of methodological flaws inherent in the study (i.e., a small sample size, the lack of long-term follow-up, and the lack of a control group).

In the second study, Grizenko et al. (1993) attempted to correct the methodological flaws inherent in the previous study by including a larger sample size, follow-up at 6 months, and a control group. The purpose of this study was to evaluate the effectiveness of a multimodal day treatment program with a psychodynamic orientation for children with disruptive behavior problems (see Grizenko & Sayegh, 1990, for a description of the program). A total of 30 children, assigned to day treatment or a waiting list (the control group), were assessed using standardized questionnaires measuring behavioral, self-perception, peer relationship, and family and academic variables. Results revealed that the treatment group showed significantly greater improvements on measures of behavior and self-perception. At 6-month follow-up, findings indicated that children in the treatment group had improved over time on all measures except academics. The authors concluded that, when compared with a control group, those children receiving day treatment services produced greater gains on the measures and that these treatment gains were maintained at follow-up.

EMERGING MODELS WITHIN SCHOOLS
It should be noted that yet another approach to mental health service delivery appears to be emerging that falls under the umbrella of day treatment. The initiation of interagency systems of care that promote the more effective use of natural settings (e.g., the school) offers a different perspective of day treatment (Lucille Eber, personal communication, February 14, 1994). One example of such an approach is the Wrap-Around Project (WRAP) being carried out by the La Grange Area Department of Special Education in Illinois and supported through a grant from the U.S. Department of Special Education (see Eber & Osuch, 1995; Eber & Stieper, 1994). Based on the premise that schools can serve as a catalyst for creating system change by creating a network of community resources for youth with emotional and behavioral disorders, the WrapAround in Schools (WAIS) model began in 1993 in three schools. The program focuses on the formation of a system that improves coordination of resources to create individualized support networks that are "wrapped" around youth and families in natural settings, such as the home,

school, and community. Evaluation of student and family outcomes, teacher perceptions, and system change indicators currently is under way. Promising initial results have been found for a sample of 25 students (see Eber & Osuch, 1995).

Yet another school-based initiative is the Vanderbilt University School-Based Counseling Evaluation Project (Catron & Weiss, 1994), a mental health services program for children from socioeconomically disadvantaged backgrounds. Established in 1990, the program is based on a collaborative, primary care model with school-based mental health clinicians providing a range of interventions and services including psychotherapy, parent skill training and education, consultative services to staff and faculty, community liaison, and case management. An evaluation of the program began in 1993 to investigate the efficacy of the program compared with traditional community-based services in such areas as early identification; service accessibility and utilization; prevention of more costly and more restrictive placements; and emotional, behavioral, and academic functioning of the students. Preliminary results have indicated that the presence of a school-based mental health program can increase service accessibility and utilization for the target population (see Catron & Weiss, 1994, for an overview of the project and preliminary results).

Another school-based mental health program is the Intensive Day Treatment (IDT), which provides a 30-day transitional educational and treatment program to youth in crisis as well as those making the transition into the community after hospitalization or residential placement (Kutok, Cox-Gerlock, Bilboa, & Kaplan, 1995). By involving the child, family, and school, the program seeks to support the child in the community and to gradually move the child back into his or her home school. Following a referral, a screening/evaluation session is held and the student is admitted to IDT for a time-limited length of stay. Both mental health and educational professionals constitute the IDT staff. The mental health staff provides clinical assessment; crisis stabilization; individual, group, and family therapy; psychopharmacology; service coordination; advocacy; and comprehensive discharge planning services. Educational personnel implement the academic assignments of the student's home school and assist students in meeting their academic objectives. Since its beginning in 1990, IDT has admitted 237 students, 81% for crisis stabilization and 19% for assisting in the youth's transition into the community. Of the 185 students discharged from the program, 78% met treatment and educational goals and had improved at discharge. A total of 13% did not meet their goals and did not improve at discharge, 6% were hospitalized, and 2% were discharged against medical advice. For all students discharged from the IDT program, 88% were reintegrated into a community school. At 30 days postdischarge, a follow-up of 109 youth who had improved at discharge indicated that 88% had maintained improvement and 12% required a new educational and/or mental health treatment plan. None of the youth were readmitted to IDT during the follow-up period. A 90-day follow-up of 59 youth who had improved at discharge revealed that 75% had maintained improvement, 17% required a new educational and/or mental health treatment plan, and 8% had been readmitted to IDT. Furthermore, the per-pupil cost for the IDT program is at least one third the cost of longer-term programs.

CONCLUSIONS AND FUTURE RESEARCH NEEDS

Based on this literature review, it appears evident that the features of day treatment vary widely across a number of variables. The programs described above represent a wide assortment of treatment settings, populations, treatment approaches, theoretical orientations, and program components. Because of the wide variability among program models, it is not possible to make conclusive statements regarding which program models of day treatment are the most effective in promoting behavioral and emotional adjustment. Furthermore, it is not yet clear who benefits from day treatment.

Although firm conclusions may not be drawn, three tentative conclusions appear to be suggested in the research contained within this review. First, the family plays a significant role in the child's outcomes after day treatment services. A number of studies found that family motivation, family involvement, and family stability during and after treatment were related to successful outcomes (see Cohen, Kolers, & Bradley, 1987; Gabel & Finn, 1986; Sack et al., 1987). Second, day treatment services may be effective for a limited population of children. Most studies found that treatment gains were less likely for children with severe behavior problems than for those with other disabilities (see Cohen, Bradley, & Kolers, 1987; Gabel et al., 1988; Grizenko & Sayegh, 1990; Sack et al., 1987; Sayegh & Grizenko, 1991). Finally, based on a small number of studies that looked at this variable, evidence seems to suggest that treatment gains have not generalized to mainstreamed school settings. For instance, Kosturn et al. (1990) found no significant change in classroom behavior after treatment. Grizenko and Sayegh (1990) found that parents reported greater improvements in behavior than did teachers or therapists. Furthermore, the findings of the study conducted by Grizenko et al. (1993) revealed that children receiving services through a multimodal day treatment program had improved on all outcome measures with the exception of academics. The implementation of school-based models of mental health service programs, such as those described above, may lead to improved outcomes in the school setting. Again, these conclusions are tentative, and further research is clearly needed.

Despite the wide variability in the features of day treatment programs and the difficulty in making conclusive statements about effectiveness, it appears that day treatment is a promising and cost-saving approach in the treatment of some children and youth with emotional problems. Certainly, further research is needed in this area. Sayegh and Grizenko (1991) stated that future research must focus upon determining the types of children and families that benefit most from this treatment approach, the areas of functioning that are most affected by day treatment, and the components of day treatment that are most effective. In addition, studies must utilize more stringent experimental designs, implement more sophisticated statistical analyses, incorporate the use of control groups, establish clearly defined outcome criteria, and utilize standardized assessment instruments (Sayegh & Grizenko, 1991; Zimet & Farley, 1985). More data are also needed on comparisons of cost and outcomes for residential treatment and day treatment (Steve Forness, personal communication, January 28, 1994).

REFERENCES

Baenen, R.S., Parris Stephens, M.A., & Glenwick, D.S. (1986). Outcome in psychoeducational day school programs: A review. *American Journal of Orthopsychiatry, 56*(2), 263–270.

Burns, B.J., & Friedman, R.M. (1990). Examining the research base for child mental health services and policy. *Journal of Mental Health Administration, 17*(1), 87–98.

Catron, T., & Weiss, B. (1994). The Vanderbilt school-based counseling program: An interagency, primary-care model of mental health services. *Journal of Emotional and Behavioral Disorders, 2*(4), 247–253.

Cohen, N.J., Bradley, S., & Kolers, N. (1987). Outcome evaluation of a therapeutic day treatment program for delayed and disturbed preschoolers. *Journal of the American Academy of Child and Adolescent Psychiatry, 26*(5), 687–693.

Cohen, N.J., Kolers, N., & Bradley, S. (1987). Predictors of the outcome of treatment in a therapeutic preschool. *Journal of the American Academy of Child and Adolescent Psychiatry, 26*(6), 829–833.

Eber, L., & Osuch, R. (1995). Bringing the wraparound approach to school: A model for inclusion. In C.J. Liberton, K. Kutash, & R.M. Friedman (Eds.), *The 7th Annual Research Conference Proceedings, A System of Care for Children's Mental Health: Expanding the Research Base* (pp. 143–151). Tampa: University of South Florida, Florida Mental Health Institute, Research and Training Center for Children's Mental Health.

Eber, L., & Stieper, C. (1994). Interagency collaboration through a school-based wraparound approach: A systems analysis summary of Project WRAP. In C.J. Liberton, K. Kutash, & R.M. Friedman (Eds.), *The 6th Annual Research Conference Proceedings, A System of Care for Children's Mental Health: Expanding the Research Base* (pp. 215–223). Tampa: University of South Florida, Florida Mental Health Institute, Research and Training Center for Children's Mental Health.

Gabel, S., & Finn, M. (1986). Outcome in children's day-treatment programs: Review of the literature and recommendations for future research. *International Journal of Partial Hospitalization, 3*(4), 261–271.

Gabel, S., Finn, M., & Ahmad, A. (1988). Day treatment outcome with severely disturbed children. *Journal of the American Academy of Child and Adolescent Psychiatry, 27*(4), 479–482.

Grizenko, N., & Papineau, D. (1992). A comparison of the cost-effectiveness of day treatment and residential treatment for children with severe behavior problems. *Canadian Journal of Psychiatry, 37*(6), 393–400.

Grizenko, N., Papineau, D., & Sayegh, L. (1993). Effectiveness of a multimodal day treatment program for children with disruptive behavior problems. *Journal of the American Academy of Child and Adolescent Psychiatry, 32*(1), 127–134.

Grizenko, N., & Sayegh, L. (1990). Evaluation of the effectiveness of a psychodynamically oriented day treatment program for children with behavior problems: A pilot study. *Canadian Journal of Psychiatry, 35*, 519–525.

Kiser, L.J., Ackerman, B.J., & Pruitt, D.B. (1987). A comparison of intensive psychiatric services for children and adolescents: Cost of day treatment versus hospitalization. *International Journal of Partial Hospitalization*, 4(1), 17–27.

Kosturn, C., Brown, N.L., & Brown, R.M. (1990). Day treatment and the behavior of emotionally disturbed children. *Journal of Social Behavior and Personality*, 5(6), 671–682.

Kutok, B., Cox-Gerlock, B., Bilboa, E., & Kaplan, S. (1995). Intensive day treatment: A short-term and transition program for children and adolescents in acute emotional crisis. In C.J. Liberton, K. Kutash, & R.M. Friedman (Eds.), *The 7th Annual Research Conference Proceedings, A System of Care for Children's Mental Health: Expanding the Research Base* (pp. 173–175). Tampa: University of South Florida, Florida Mental Health Institute, Research and Training Center for Children's Mental Health.

LeCroy, C.W., & Ashford, J.B. (1992). Children's mental health: Current findings and research directions. *Social Work Research & Abstracts*, 28(1), 13–20.

Orchard, J.M., & MacLeod, R.J. (1990). Adolescent day program: A two year retrospective review. *Canadian Journal of Psychiatry*, 35(6), 554–556.

Parker, S., & Knoll, J.L. (1990). Partial hospitalization: An update. *American Journal of Psychiatry*, 147(2), 156–160.

Research and Training Center for Children's Mental Health. (1985–1986). Day treatment. *Update*, 1(2).

Sack, W.H., Mason, R., & Collins, R. (1987). A long-term follow-up study of a children's psychiatric day treatment center. *Child Psychiatry and Human Development*, 18(1), 58–68.

Sayegh, L., & Grizenko, N. (1991). Studies of the effectiveness of day treatment programs for children. *Canadian Journal of Psychiatry*, 36(4), 246–253.

Stroul, B.A., & Friedman, R.M. (1986). *A system of care for children and youth with severe emotional disturbances* (rev. ed.). Washington, DC: Georgetown University Child Development Center, National Assistance Center for Children's Mental Health.

Topp, D.B. (1991). Beyond the continuum of care: Conceptualizing day treatment for children and youth. *Community Mental Health Journal*, 27(2), 105–113.

Tuma, J.M. (1989). Mental health services for children: The state of the art. *American Psychologist*, 44(2), 188–199.

Zimet, S.G., & Farley, G.K. (1985). Day treatment for children in the United States. *Journal of the American Academy of Child Psychiatry*, 24(6), 732–738.

CHAPTER 3

Home-Based Services

Home-based services (Burns & Friedman, 1990), also commonly referred to as family preservation services, in-home services, family-centered services, family-based services, or intensive family services (Anders-Cibik, Zarski, Cleminshaw, & Greenbank, 1990; Cole & Duva, 1990), is an approach to the treatment of children and families that was first developed in the 1970s. Although a number of both public and private child-serving agencies are involved in providing home-based services, most programs share similar characteristics. On the basis of descriptions set forth in the literature, Stroul and Goldman (1990) have listed the common features of home-based services as follows:

1. The intervention is delivered primarily in the family's home.
2. Services are family focused, and the family is considered the client.
3. Services have an "ecological" perspective and involve working in collaboration with the community to access and coordinate community supports and services.
4. Service programs are committed to family preservation and reunification unless there is evidence that the safety of the child is jeopardized.
5. Service delivery hours are flexible in order to meet the needs of the families, and 24-hour crisis intervention services are provided.
6. Services are multifaceted and include counseling, skill training, and assisting the family in obtaining and coordinating needed services, resources, and supports.
7. Services vary along a continuum of intensity and duration based upon the goals of the program and needs of the family.

8. Staff have small caseloads (two to three families), which permit them to work in an active and intense manner with each family.
9. The relationship between the home-based worker and the family is uniquely close, intense, and personal.
10. Programs are committed to empowering families, instilling hope in families, and assisting families in setting and achieving personal goals and priorities.

As noted, home-based services vary with regard to service intensity and duration. Family preservation represents one type of service under the rubric of home-based services. Family preservation services are defined as "short term, in-home, intensive, crisis intervention services" having an ecological perspective and a family-based focus (Yelton, 1991, p. 7). Thus, family preservation services tend to be of short duration (ranging from 1 to 3 months), but are highly intensive (10–20 or more hours per week). Services are provided to families in which a child is at imminent risk for placement in a more restrictive setting due to child abuse, neglect, juvenile delinquency, status offenses, emotional problems, or school difficulties (Forsythe, 1992) and are usually rendered only when other interventions have proven unsuccessful (Cole & Duva, 1990). The Child Welfare League of America (1989) has established a set of standards for the delivery of family preservation services. These standards provide a thorough description of the goals of family preservation programs that are designed to strengthen and preserve families with children.

Most family preservation services have three primary goals: 1) to preserve the integrity of the family and to prevent the unnecessary placement of children in substitute care while simultaneously ensuring the safety of the child, 2) to develop an ongoing community support system by linking the family with appropriate community agencies and individuals, and 3) to increase the coping skills of the family and its capacity to function effectively in the community (Stroul & Goldman, 1990). In addition, family preservation services are used to assist children already in placements to reunify with their families (Anders-Cibik et al., 1990; Stroul & Goldman, 1990).

There has been a significant increase in the number of family preservation programs since the mid-1980s (National Resource Center on Family-Based Services, 1991). This growth has been attributed to a number of factors:

1. The increasing number of children in out-of-home placements and dissatisfaction with these placements, especially foster care
2. An increased focus on family integrity and the importance of the parent-child relationship
3. The move toward an ecological perspective in the provision of treatment rather than an individualistic perspective
4. The establishment of public policy mandates (e.g., Adoption Assistance and Child Welfare Act of 1980; PL 96-272) that strive to preserve families
5. The search for less expensive alternatives to care (Whittaker & Tracy, 1990)

FUNDING AND COST COMPARISONS

Funding

Until the passage of the Omnibus Budget Reconciliation Act of 1993 (PL 103-66), there was no federal funding stream specifically targeted for family preservation programs (Cole & Duva, 1990). Signed into law in August 1993, this act provided new federal funding for family preservation services. Over a 5-year period, one billion dollars in child welfare funds will be provided to states for a variety of early intervention and prevention services with the intent of strengthening, preserving, supporting, and/or reunifying troubled, at-risk children and their families. In the past, most states have redirected funds to implement pilot projects or family preservation services on a statewide basis. A descriptive study of community-based services for children and adolescents with serious emotional disorders found that state government represented the major funding source for the provision of home-based programs, and the state mental health department represented the second most frequent source of funding (Stroul & Goldman, 1990). The practice of shared financing among various child-serving agencies represents yet another commonly used funding approach. Family preservation services increasingly are being funded through collaborations among departments of mental health, child welfare, and, at times, juvenile justice (Knitzer & Yelton, 1990).

Costs

The reported costs of providing home-based services vary widely due to differences in intensity and duration of programs, variations in staffing patterns and salaries, and differences in accounting and costing approaches (Hutchinson, 1982). In a comparison of home-based services and out-of-home placements, Polsky (1986) estimated the annual cost per child of home-based services as ranging from $3,000 to $5,000, whereas the annual cost per child of foster care placement was reported at $5,000, group home placement at $10,000, detention at $20,000, residential treatment center placement at $30,000, and psychiatric hospitalization at $40,000. Furthermore, cost differentials are substantially greater when one considers that children are often in out-of-home placements for more than 1 year.

Kinney, Haapala, and Booth (1991) reported the cost savings of the Homebuilders model of family preservation for sites in Washington State and the Bronx, New York. During 1989 in Washington State, the cost of Homebuilders averaged $2,700 per child for those deemed appropriate for placement. A comparison of the difference between the cost of Homebuilders and various out-of-home placements in Washington State illustrated the cost savings. For example, the total cost of Homebuilders for 60 children was $162,200/year ($2,700/child); the cost of foster care for the same number of children was estimated to be $468,780/year ($7,813/child).

When compared with other more restrictive placements, such as residential treatment centers and psychiatric hospitalization, the use of family preservation services resulted in substantially greater cost savings. An analysis of the initial results of the Bronx Project revealed that the cost for Homebuilders services for the first 6 months was $211,892 for all children. This estimated cost is $2,306,048 *less* than the average cost of out-of-home placement (e.g., psychiatric hospital, residential treatment center) for the same number of children.

An examination of the cost savings of the Families First program in Michigan, compared with traditional foster care services, was conducted over a 6-month evaluation period (Michigan Department of Social Services, 1993). Of the 626 families referred to Families First during this 6-month period, 96% of the families were deemed by child protective service workers as having children at risk of out-of-home placement. Assuming that this estimate was correct, the prevention of foster care placement for 96% of the children referred to Families First over the program's 3-year period (n = 6,656) could have saved the state more than $55,000,000 for the first year after the family preservation intervention. It should be noted that, due to the low cost of the Families First program, cost savings would remain substantial even if a more conservative estimate of the percentage of children at risk for placement was used.

A financial analysis was also conducted to determine the financial savings achieved through utilization of the Family Ties program operated by the New York City Department of Juvenile Justice (New York City Department of Juvenile Justice, 1993). The average cost per year for placement in the New York State Division for Youth facility is about $70,000/child. This cost is distributed equally between the city of New York and the state of New York. The Family Ties program achieved a total savings of $11,043,318 in placement costs from FY 1989 through the first half of FY 1992.

The cost savings of family preservation and family reunification services has been supported in other studies as well (see Berry, 1992; Henggeler, Melton, & Smith, 1992; Woodworth, Hyde, Jordan, & Burchard, 1994). On the basis of these and other studies, it appears that family preservation services result in savings in comparison with out-of-home placements, especially residential placement settings.

According to K. Wells (personal communication, February 8, 1994), methodologies used to determine the cost savings of family preservation services are fraught with difficulties and must be viewed with caution. For example, most cost determinations do not include the cost of followup services that accompany family preservation services. To be accurate, all related services used by families during treatment and after service termination must be considered.

EFFECTIVENESS AND OUTCOME RESEARCH

The developers of family preservation services have led the way in conducting research to evaluate the effectiveness of this approach. Early evaluations of family preservation services revealed generally positive results; however, these investigations have been criticized for using a single-outcome criterion (i.e., the avoidance of out-of-home placement), small sample sizes, and methodological flaws (see Hinckley & Ellis, 1985; Kinney, Madsen, Fleming, & Haapala, 1977). Studies in the 1990s have attempted to address these criticisms by examining multiple treatment outcomes, exploring correlates of treatment success and failure, and employing experimental and quasi-experimental research designs (e.g., Wells & Biegel, 1991). The most frequently cited literature examining the effectiveness of family preservation services is summarized in this section.

Homebuilders

The Homebuilders program, established in 1974 in Tacoma, Washington, is perhaps the best known of the family preservation programs and has served as a model for the establishment of several similar programs across the country. Early reports of the Homebuilders program indicated a success rate of greater than 90%; that is, less than 10% of the children who received family preservation services were placed outside the home (Kinney et al., 1977).

A major study was conducted by Fraser, Pecora, and Haapala (1988) to evaluate the Homebuilders program and to compare it with a similar program in Utah. This study examined the initial outcomes for 453 families and included a 12-month follow-up for 263 families. Overall, more than 70% of the families remained intact at service termination. At the 12-month follow-up, approximately 66% of the Homebuilders families and over 56% of the Utah families remained intact. Those families who remained together also received improved ratings on a variety of measures, including school adjustment, delinquent behavior, behavior at home, parenting and supervision of children, parental knowledge about child care, and parental attitudes toward placement.

Pecora, Fraser, and Haapala (1991, 1992) examined six intensive family preservation programs and collected pretest–posttest data from families receiving family preservation services in Utah (two sites) and Washington State (four sites). For the families in Utah, almost 91% remained intact; and for families in Washington State, the rate was almost 94% at service termination. On the average, 93% of the at-risk children who received intensive family preservation services remained with their families or relatives at termination. A total of four children were placed with relatives at or before termination of services. When placement with relatives was considered a service failure, the treatment success rate was 92.3% for children at all sites. For the cases in Utah, the rate was 89.5%, and the rate for Washington cases was 93.4%.

Placement prevention rates for the 12-month follow-up group ($n = 263$ families) indicated that treatment gains had declined over time. Of the 342 children who were followed for 12 months after receiving family preservation services, 67% remained with their families or relatives throughout the year. The placement rates of a small comparison group (26 Utah families who had been referred for family preservation services, but instead received traditional services) were compared with those in the treatment group. The out-of-home placement rate was higher for those in the comparison group (traditional services) than for those in the treatment group (family preservation services). The out-of-home placement rate for the comparison group was almost twice that of the treatment group when compared at 12 months (85% and 44%, respectively).

In addition, a more stringent analysis was conducted to compare the treatment success of the Utah comparison group cases with a matched set of cases receiving intensive family preservation services. Cases in the comparison group and the experimental group were matched on the following characteristics: the child's race, gender, school attendance, suspected or substantiated substance abuse, disability status, and previous inpatient treatment history as well as family income, family structure, and size of household. For the subset of matched treatment cases receiving intensive family preservation services, the placement rate was 44%. This rate was significantly lower than the placement rate for comparison group cases (85%).

In 1987, a Homebuilders program was established in the Bronx, New York. The program served children who were abused and neglected. Data collected from May 1987 through August 1988 represented 58 families with 101 children at risk of placement. Approximately 13% of the children were in "official placement" (placement settings such as foster care, group care, residential treatment, or hospitalization as opposed to placement with relatives) 3 months after termination of Homebuilders services (Kinney et al., 1991).

Hennepin County, Minnesota
The Center for the Study of Youth Policy at the University of Minnesota conducted an evaluation of a family preservation pilot program established in 1985 (AuClaire & Schwartz, 1986; Schwartz, AuClaire, & Harris, 1991). Families were deemed eligible for participation in the study if they had been approved previously for a home-based placement by both a supervisor and a program manager. A comparison group (n = 58) was composed of a randomly selected sample of adolescents who were eligible to receive home-based services but could not be served because the pilot program was full. The use of all residential placements by subjects was documented over a 12- to 16-month period. Results revealed that youth receiving family preservation services (n = 55) experienced fewer out-of-home placements (56%) than did those in the comparison group (91%). *However, the groups did not differ significantly with regard to the incidence of placement when out-of-home placements such as living with extended family or friends was included.* Those in the treatment group experienced fewer days in placement (2,368) in comparison with the control group (3,803). The two groups did *not* differ in the average number of placements; however, those receiving home-based services were placed in less restrictive settings.

Maryland
Pearson, Masnyk, and King (1987) conducted a preliminary evaluation of the Intensive Family Services pilot project in

Maryland. Evaluation data from 1984 revealed that only 10% of the families receiving services experienced a placement. Furthermore, those counties in which the Intensive Family Services project was implemented experienced a substantially greater decline in the use of foster care than did counties in which such services were not available. A more extensive study conducted the following year found that families receiving intensive family services experienced fewer placements and had significantly lower scores on measures of risk to the child compared with families who received traditional services.

California

In 1984 the California legislature authorized a bill to fund eight intensive home-based service projects with the purpose of preventing foster care placement and lowering the subsequent abuse or neglect of children under the age of 14. A 3-year study was conducted by W. R. McDonald and Associates, Inc. to evaluate the effectiveness of these programs (see McDonald & Associates, Inc. 1990; Yuan, McDonald, Wheeler, Struckman-Johnson, & Rivest, 1990). During the third year of the projects, an investigation was carried out that examined the functioning of families with one or more children at risk of out-of-home placement. More specifically, the study compared the number of placements for families receiving services from five intensive family preservation service projects across California (the treatment group) with that for a group of families receiving traditional services (the control group). Families were randomly assigned to either the treatment condition ($n = 152$) or the control condition ($n = 152$). Placement data were obtained from time of referral to 8 months after the referral. Results led to the following six conclusions:

1. No significant differences were found in the proportions of treatment and control families who experienced a placement.
2. No significant differences were observed in the number of treatment and control families who were investigated for abuse and/or neglect following their inclusion in the study.

3. No significant differences were observed between the treatment and control groups in the number of days spent in placement.
4. Significant differences were found between the treatment and control groups in the number of children placed within two months of referral.
5. Children in the treatment and control groups experienced an equal number of placement incidents.
6. Placement days with relatives and foster families "accounted for 91.2 percent of all placement days and 81.9 percent of [all] the [placed] children in the . . . control groups or 85.4 percent of all placement days and 72.8 percent of [all] of the [placed] children in the . . . experimental group" (McDonald & Associates, 1990, p. 617).

A number of problems, such as high staff turnover rate and difficulty getting referrals from child protective services, were experienced throughout the 3-year project. The evaluation report provides extensive explanations of the difficulties experienced by the project sites (see Yuan et al., 1990).

New Jersey
Using an experimental design, Feldman (1991) evaluated the effectiveness of five intensive family preservation programs. Families deemed eligible to receive family preservation services were randomly assigned to either the experimental group (family preservation services, $n = 96$) or the control group (traditional services, $n = 87$) in one of four New Jersey counties. Data were collected on out-of-home placement, family functioning, and family characteristics for up to 1 year after service termination. Results revealed that early in the treatment program (from 1 to 9 months) significantly fewer children in the treatment group experienced out-of-home placements; however, these differences in placement rates dissipated by the 12th month of treatment. Furthermore, families in the treatment group generally failed to improve on measures of family functioning as compared with those in the control group.

Iowa
Thieman and Dall (1992) reported the results of the evaluation of a statewide family preservation program in Iowa,

modeled after Homebuilders. The purposes of the study were to assess changes in family functioning through a pretest–posttest assessment as measured by the Family Risk Scales (see Magura, Moses, & Jones, 1987) and to examine the validity of these scales as a predictor of risk for foster care placement. At the time of publication of the report, data had been collected on approximately 1,500 families. Data collection was limited to families who had been served during 1990–1991, a total of 995 families. Assessment of the child's risk for out-of-home placement was obtained using the Family Risk Scales. Risk for out-of-home placement was based on three factors: parent-centered risk, child-centered risk, and economic risk. Pretest scores were used to divide the families into categories of higher risk (Group 1) or lower risk (Group 2) for out-of-home placement. Results indicated that the instrument was not useful in predicting out-of-home placement of children at service termination and that it failed to identify the acute risk characteristics of families referred for family preservation services. Results did indicate modest, but statistically significant, increases in family functioning from initiation to termination of service for both higher- and lower-risk groups as measured by the scales; however, change was most evident for those in the higher risk group. An uncertainty regarding the effectiveness of the instrument in predicting out-of-home placement risk and the lack of a comparison group were limitations inherent in this study. Evaluation activities that address these limitations are currently under way.

Northern California

Berry (1992) conducted an evaluation of the In-Home Family Care Program, an intensive family preservation program in Northern California. Over a 3-year period, data were collected for a total of 367 cases. Measures included case outcomes, client characteristics, and service characteristics. Results revealed that only 4% of the families experienced an out-of-home placement while receiving family preservation services. A total of 6% experienced out-of-home placements within 6 months after services were terminated, and 12% of the families experienced a placement at 12-month follow-up. Thus, out-of-home placements were avoided in 88% of the families served by this program. The type of service provided was found to have an effect on treatment outcome. Concrete services such as teaching family care skills, supplemental parenting, medical care, financial services, and assistance in obtaining food were found to be associated with parents who improved their parenting skills and families that remained together after termination from the program. It appears that this program was effective in preventing foster care placement as well as in initiating lasting improvements in family functioning through providing of concrete services. Further studies are currently under way to examine the recurrence of abuse charges upon termination of services.

Texas

Leben and Smith (1992) reported the results of two intensive family intervention projects in Texas. Findings were based on data for 109 youth and families who received intensive family intervention services from August 1989 through April 1991. These two project sites served adolescents with emotional disorders who either were returning from an out-of-home placement or were at risk for removal from the family setting. Results indicated that the program was successful in avoiding an out-of-home placement during treatment for about 79% of all children. At the end of the project, about 62% of the youth had remained in the home and had not experienced an out-of-home placement. Using a 5-point rating scale, therapists or program directors rated improvement in functioning as compared with initial intake impressions. Almost 25% of the adolescents were rated by their therapists as functioning *much better*, and 33% were rated as *better*. The remaining adolescents were rated as *the same, worse,* or *much worse* at the closing of the case. Using the same rating system, therapists rated improvement in parents' functioning after service termination. About 20% of the families were rated as functioning *much better*, and about 35% were rated as functioning *better*. Follow-up information indicated that 62% of the adolescents were still living at home. Almost 60% of the families finished the "full term" of treatment, and 75% who were referred for additional outpatient counseling went at least once after completing the program.

It appears that the program was successful in avoiding out-of-home placement for the majority of adolescents in the study, although placement avoidance rates had decreased by the end of the project. Furthermore, greater than half of the adolescents and families were rated by the therapists as functioning *much better* or *better* at service termination. The findings of this study are limited by the use of a descriptive and formative design; however, a more comprehensive program evaluation is currently under way.

Michigan

In response to increased public concern over a statewide increase in cases of child abuse, neglect, and delinquency, the Michigan Department of Social Services (MDSS) created a family preservation program, Families First, designed to serve as an alternative to traditional child protective service approaches such as foster care. The program provided a range of support services on an intensive, short-term basis to families in crisis. An evaluation (Michigan Department of Social Services, 1993) was conducted to determine the program's effectiveness, as compared with foster care services, in averting out-of-home placements for children. The evaluation involved a group of children ($n = 225$) who received family preservation services through the Families First program and a matched group of children ($n = 225$) who received traditional foster care services. The study covered a 3-year period and utilized multiple data sources.

In an examination of out-of-home placement rates for the two groups, results revealed that children in the Families First program evidenced a consistently lower out-of-home placement rate at 3, 6, and 12 months after the intervention. At 3-month follow-up, out-of-home placement rates were 7% for the Families First group and 15% for the foster care group. Follow-up data at 6 months revealed out-of-home placement rates of 12% for the Families First group and 26% for the foster care group. Out-of-home placement rates at 12-month follow-up were 24% for children in the Families First group and 35% for those in foster care. Even more striking differences were noted in out-of-home placement rates for the two groups when 39 pairs of children referred as a result of delinquency and who were working toward reunification with their families were removed from the analysis. For the matched pairs of children ($N = 186$ pairs) referred because of abuse and/or neglect, respective out-of-home placement rates at 3, 6, and 12 months were 5%, 13%, and 19% for the children in the Families First group and 12%, 26%, and 36% for children who received foster care services.

Examination of Child and Family Functioning

In a study designed to examine child and family functioning after intensive family preservation services, Wells and Whittington (1993) sought to answer two important questions: 1) how well were families who received family preservation services functioning at follow-up; and 2) did family functioning improve between admission and discharge, and, if so, was improvement maintained at follow-up? A sample of 42 families was included in the analyses. A family was eligible to participate in the study if it had a child between the ages of 10 and 18 years who had been referred to the family preservation program. Data were collected from children, parents, and caseworkers at admission, discharge, and 1 year after service termination.

Sources of data included measures of family and child functioning, the resolution of problems reported at admission, and stability of the child's living situation between discharge and follow-up. Family and child functioning, as measured by three standardized instruments, was defined in terms of the promotion of family health, the elimination or reduction of parent–child conflict, and the amelioration of child behavioral problems. The resolution of admission problems was defined as the degree to which the problems reported by parents and children at admission had improved and the proportion of these problems that had been eliminated by discharge or follow-up as measured by self-report. The stability of a child's living situation between discharge and follow-up was defined as the extent to which the child remained in the home he or she was in at discharge or was scheduled to return to at discharge. The stability measure reflected the number of changes in placement between discharge and follow-up.

Follow-up results revealed that, on average, families in this program were functioning at a lower level than were a standardized sample of families (i.e., a nonclinical sample). Specifically, both children and parents reported the health of their families and their relationships with each other as more problematic and their children's behavior problems as more severe than those of the nonclinical sample. Children's behaviors and parent–child relationships were evaluated in a more negative manner by parents than by children. Evaluations of family health were similar for parents and children.

With regard to the resolution of admission problems, parents and children reported that many of the problems apparent at admission were resolved or had improved at follow-up. On average, children stated that more than 50% of the problems they had reported at admission were eliminated or resolved; and for those problems still present, children reported modest improvement since discharge. At follow-up, parents reported on average that more than one third of the problems at admission were eliminated or resolved. Parents reported modest improvement for those problems that were still present.

During the follow-up period, measures of stability indicated that the majority of children (59%) remained in the home in which they had lived at discharge. Of those who did experience placement changes, the highest percentage (47%) moved only once, 41% experienced from two to four placement changes, and the remainder (12%) experienced eight or nine moves. Results of the use of out-of-home placements between discharge and follow-up indicated that 80% of the children had no out-of-home placements, and the remaining children were placed in psychiatric hospitals, group homes, correctional facilities, residential treatment centers, foster homes, or child care institutions.

In the examination of improvements in child and family functioning over time, results revealed that, on average, the functioning of children and families improved between admission and discharge and did not decline between discharge and follow-up. A statistically significant difference was noted in children's average scores from admission (2.50) to discharge (2.30) to follow-up (2.28) as measured by the Family

Assessment Device–Version 3 (Epstein, Baldwin, & Bishop, 1983). Scores decreased from admission to discharge, but remained essentially the same from discharge to follow-up. Scores on the Child Behavior Checklist (Achenbach & Edelbrock, 1983a) and Youth Self-Report Form (Achenbach & Edelbrock, 1983b) were found to be statistically different over time, with a mean score of 73.15 at admission, 69.73 at discharge, and 62.44 at follow-up. Furthermore, no significant difference was noted between discharge and follow-up in change in admission problems because the level of improvement at discharge was maintained at follow-up.

FAMILY PRESERVATION AND HOME-BASED SERVICES WITH JUVENILE JUSTICE POPULATIONS

Haapala and Kinney (1988) reported the success of a Homebuilders program designed to avert out-of-home placement for status-offending youth who were at risk for foster care or residential placement. Participants in the study were 678 status-offending youth referred to Homebuilders. Youth and their families received family preservation services from one of four Homebuilders programs in Washington State. Placement prevention rates were gathered for youth at 12 months after they began the Homebuilders program. Of the 678 youth receiving services, 592 (87%) avoided out-of-home placement during the 12-month follow-up period. The remaining youth were placed in foster, group, or residential care. Although the results of this study are promising, findings must be viewed with caution due to the lack of a comparison group and the possible effects of additional counseling services received by the families after termination from the Homebuilders program.

South Carolina

Henggeler et al. (1992) conducted a study to examine the efficacy of a family preservation program using multisystemic family therapy (MST) in decreasing the rates of institutionalization of youthful offenders and in reducing antisocial behavior. Eighty-four juvenile offenders judged to be at risk for out-of-home placement participated in the study. Results revealed that, at 59 weeks postreferral, youth who had received family preservation services using multisystemic treatment had approximately half as many arrests as did youth who received traditional services. Recidivism rates (rates of re-arrest) were 42% for the treatment group and 62% for the comparison group. Furthermore, a composite measure of family cohesion indicated that families participating in the family preservation program experienced greater cohesion, whereas families receiving traditional services experienced decreased cohesion. A composite measure of aggression toward peers revealed that those youth in the treatment condition had a decreased level of aggression, whereas those in the control condition experienced no change in aggression as a result of treatment. These findings support the efficacy of a family preservation program using multisystemic therapy in reducing out-of-home placements and in decreasing criminal activity as compared with traditional service delivery methods.

Through a search of archival data, long-term follow-up data on re-arrest for the above sample ($N = 84$) were gathered for an average of 2.4 years postreferral (Henggeler, Melton, Smith, Schoenwald, & Hanley, 1993). Results revealed that multisystemic family preservation was more effective than traditional services in prolonging the time to re-arrest for this sample. The mean time to re-arrest for those receiving multisystemic family preservation services was about 56 weeks, whereas the mean time to re-arrest for those receiving traditional services was about 32 weeks. At 120 weeks postreferral, 39% of those in the multisystemic family preservation group had not been re-arrested, whereas 20% of those receiving traditional services had not been re-arrested.

Other controlled clinical studies have examined the effectiveness of family preservation using multisystemic treatment with adolescents having substance abuse and serious criminal behavior (see Henggeler, Schoenwald, Borduin, et al., 1994, and Henggeler, Schoenwald, Pickrel, Rowland, & Santos, 1994, for a brief review of these studies). Findings from the Missouri Delinquency Project represent the most comprehensive and extensive evaluation of family preservation using MST. Chronic juvenile offenders ($N = 200$) were randomly assigned to either a group that received

MST or a group that received individual therapy. In addition to recidivism data for 4 years after treatment, pretest–posttest self-report and observational measures were collected to assess individual, peer, and family functioning. Observational measures revealed that families who received MST exhibited more supportiveness and less conflict/hostility in mother–adolescent, father–adolescent, and mother–father relations compared with those families in the individual therapy condition. Those in the MST group also reported more family cohesion and adaptability. Adolescents in the MST group displayed significantly fewer behavior problems after treatment, and parents reported less symptomatology. Follow-up data at 4 years indicated that recidivism rates were 22% (MST group) and 71% (individual therapy) for those who completed therapy. Of those who were re-arrested, those in the MST group were arrested less often and for less serious crimes than were those in the comparison group.

Another randomized controlled study examining the effectiveness of family preservation using MST was conducted in Charleston, South Carolina. Adolescents ($N = 112$) exhibiting both substance abuse and delinquency problems were randomly assigned to either the MST group or the usual services group. A battery of assessment devices were administered at pretreatment, at posttreatment, and at 6- and 12-month follow-up periods. Preliminary results from 20 cases revealed that the MST group experienced more gains in abstinence from substance abuse and delinquency resulting in decreased institutionalization as compared with the usual services group (Henggeler, Schoenwald, Borduin, et al., 1994).

City of New York
The New York City Department of Juvenile Justice was the first juvenile justice agency in the nation to implement a placement diversion program (Family Ties) based on the Homebuilders model of family preservation (Collier & Hill, 1993). The primary objective of the program was to prevent the unnecessary placement of adjudicated juvenile delinquents by directly intervening in the youths' life and assisting with problem areas that contributed to the delinquency.

A quasi-experimental design was employed to measure outcome differences between youth in the Family Ties program and a group of juveniles not served by the program. Primary outcome measures included rates of re-arrest, reconviction, and reincarceration for the year after release from the Family Ties program or, for those in the comparison group, from the state youth facility. Positive behavior changes exhibited by program youths also were used to assess outcome. Former program youth ($n = 93$) were randomly selected for inclusion in the study. Of that number, 57% ($n = 40$ families) consented to an interview. The comparison group was comprised of randomly selected juvenile delinquents ($n = 40$) who were adjudicated in family court and placed in a state youth facility. Groups were found to be comparable in background and at-risk variables and had been in the community about the same length of time (1 year) before follow-up.

Results indicated that the program was able to avert from placement an average of 65% of the youth received through court referrals. This placement aversion rate falls within the normative range for similar family preservation programs. For youth and families participating in the program during 1991–1992, 6-month data indicated that approximately 8 in 10 youth remained uninvolved with the juvenile justice system. No significant difference was noted between 6- and 12-month follow-up. Rates of reinvolvement were significantly lower for those in the Family Ties program than for the comparison group. For those in the program, the rate of re-arrest was 20%, and reconviction and reincarceration rates were each 18%. For the comparison group, the rate of re-arrest was 42% and the rates of reconviction and reincarceration were 40% each. As another measure of outcome, the evaluation focused on the amount of placement time saved as a result of the Family Ties program. In 1992, on average, the program averted almost 6 weeks of placement time during the program and nearly 10 months after participation in the program. For results on the program's model and process, see Collier and Hill (1993).

FAMILY REUNIFICATION SERVCIES

Utah

Rather than focusing on the use of family preservation as a way of preventing out-of-home placements, Walton, Fraser,

Lewis, Pecora, and Walton (1993) examined the effectiveness of family preservation services in reunifying children with their families. This Utah study utilized a posttest-only experimental design. Families were randomly selected from a computer-generated list of children in out-of-home care. Each family was randomly assigned to either the treatment or control group. The treatment condition comprised a group of families (n = 57) who received family preservation services, whereas those in the control condition consisted of families (n = 53) who received traditional family foster care reunification services. Data were collected at the beginning and end of the 3-month treatment period.

Findings revealed that at the end of the 90-day treatment period, 93% of the families in the treatment group were reunited, compared with only 28.3% of the families in the control group. Data at 6 months revealed a reverse in the trend apparent at the end of the treatment period in that some of the children in the treatment group had returned to an out-of-home placement, whereas more of the children in the control group had been reunited with their families. Of the 53 children in the treatment group who were living at home at the end of the treatment period, 40 (70% of the total treatment group) remained in the home 6 months later. During this time, an additional 7 children in the control group returned home, resulting in a total of 22 (41.5%) living at home. Data collected at 12 months after the termination of services revealed that 43 (75.4%) of the children in the treatment group were in their homes, compared with 26 (49%) of the children in the control group. Furthermore, those receiving family preservation services spent significantly more days living at home during the 90-day treatment period and follow-up periods than did those receiving traditional services.

New England
Fein and Staff (1993) reported the findings from the first 2 years of a 3-year demonstration project in New England. In 1989, Casey Family Services, a private child welfare agency, expanded its services to include three reunification programs located in Connecticut, Maine, and Vermont. These reunification programs were designed to serve children placed in

state family or group foster care due to abuse or neglect and who had a permanency plan that called for reunification with the biological family.

During the first 2 years of the demonstration project, 110 children (47 families) were served by the program. Children ($N = 68$) who had received services for 6 or more months were the focus of the current analyses. During the first 2 years, 26 of the children (38%) had been reunited with their biological families. Of those 68 children, 13 (19%) were at home and still receiving services, 6 (9%) were at home and their case had been closed, and 7 (10%) were returned to out-of-home care; the remaining 42 children (62%) were not reunified (they were working toward reunification, moving toward another permanency plan, or not reunified–case closed). Thus, 19 of the 26 unified children (28% of the total 68) remained reunified with their families by the end of the second year of the project.

Baltimore, Maryland

Woodworth et al. (1994) presented the findings of two initial studies of the Family Preservation Initiative of Baltimore City, Inc. (FPI), founded in January 1991. Based on a wraparound care model approach for the provision of family reunification services, this initiative was designed to return children from out-of-state placements, divert inappropriate out-of-home and out-of-state placements, and redirect funding streams from out-of-home placements to community-based placements.

Study 1 examined the effectiveness of FPI services and the use of the principles of wraparound services by evaluating the outcomes of youth returned and diverted from out-of-home placements. Participants in the study included all youth returned and diverted from out-of-state care by July 1, 1993. Information was gathered about each youth's history and placement changes. Updated information was collected on a monthly basis. The Restrictiveness of Living Environments Scale (ROLES) (Hawkins, Almeida, Fabry, & Reitz, 1992) was used to provide an index of the restrictiveness level of residential placements. Data on adjustment behaviors (e.g., school suspensions, psychiatric hospitalizations, attempted suicides, delinquent arrests) were gathered to monitor the progress of the youth.

Prior to entering FPI service, 20% of the youth were in placements having a restrictiveness level of 5.5 (group home level care) or less. At the end of 1993, the percentage of youth in placements having a restrictive level of 5.5 or less had risen to 82%. With regard to the number of residential placements while in FPI care, the majority of youth (65%) had only one placement, 30% had two to four placements, and 5% had five to seven placements. In terms of school placement, 65% had only one placement, 26% had two placements, and 19% had three placements. The following results were obtained for the occurrence of adjustment behaviors: 30% exhibited none of the behaviors, 29% experienced school suspensions, 21% experienced psychiatric hospitalizations, 6% attempted suicide, and 14% experienced delinquent arrests. Parent and youth satisfaction measures of services and programs were obtained by phone. On a scale of 1 (very dissatisfied) to 5 (very satisfied), parents reported an overall mean rating of 3.5 on measures of satisfaction with services, and youth reported an overall mean rating of 3.9. With regard to satisfaction with various program components, parents had an overall mean rating of 3.8, and youth had an overall mean score of 3.5.

Study 2 examined the effectiveness of FPI services specifically for youth returned from out-of-state placement. Data were gathered for a sample of youth ($N = 30$) who had been returned from out-of-state placement and who had received FPI services for at least 6 months. Results suggested that FPI's methods of returning youth from out-of-state placements assisted them in maintaining less restrictive placements than before out-of-state placement. Those who returned from out-of-state placements revealed a decrease in both level of restrictiveness and number of placements. Furthermore, psychiatric hospitalization was found to be the best predictor of level of restrictiveness after out-of-state placement. That is, youth with a greater number of psychiatric hospitalizations upon return from out-of-state placements were more likely to be placed in more restrictive environments. However, increased length of out-of-state placement was not found to be related to higher levels of restrictiveness upon return to the state. A second analysis revealed that youth in more restrictive placements prior to leaving the state spent a longer amount of time in out-of-state placements.

CONCLUSIONS AND FUTURE RESEARCH NEEDS

Based on the studies included in this review, it appears that family preservation services have been effective in averting placement of a high percentage of children. At service termination, the percentage of children remaining with their families ranged from about 70% to 96% (see Table 3.1). Most studies, however, did not utilize a control or comparison group. The percentage of children averted from placement tended to decrease at follow-up. However, percentages were greater for those receiving family preservation services at follow-up than for those in comparison or control groups.

Few studies examined outcome measures other than placement prevention rates. Of the 18 studies reviewed, only 2 explored the effects of family preservation services on child or family functioning. Thieman and Dall (1992) found a statistically significant increase in family functioning from admission to termination for those receiving family preservation services. Wells and Whittington (1993) found that family functioning improved between admission and discharge, with no decline apparent between discharge and follow-up. Many of the problems present at admission had been resolved or had improved. Almost 60% of the children had remained in the home in which they lived at discharge.

Similar trends were apparent in the studies that examined the use of family preservation services in reunifying families—that is, reuniting children already in out-of-home placements with their families. Whereas the percentage of children reunified was greater for those in the treatment compared with the control groups, those percentages decreased as the amount of time from discharge increased. In an examination of outcomes other than rate of placement prevention, Woodworth et al. (1994) found that restrictiveness of placements was less during the period after 6 months of family preservation services than during the period prior to out-of-state placement.

Table 3.1. Summary of studies evaluating family preservation and family reunification services

	Percentage of children with family and other notable outcomes						
	At service termination		At 12-month follow-up		At other frequencies of follow-up		Sample size
Authors	Treatment	Control	Treatment	Control	Treatment	Control	
Haapala & Kinney (1988)[a]	—	—	87%	—	—	—	N = 678 status offenders
Fraser, Pecora, & Haapala (1988)	>70%	—	66% (WA)[b] 56% (UT)[b]	—	—	—	N = 453 families at service termination; N = 263 families at 12-month follow-up
Pecora, Fraser, & Haapala (1991, 1992)	93%[c]	—	56%	15%	—	—	N = 581 children initially; N = 263 families at 12-month follow-up; n = 26 families in control group at 12-month follow-up
Kinney, Haapala, & Booth (1991)	87%[d]	—	—	—	—	—	N = 58 families (101 children)
AuClaire & Schwartz (1986); Schwartz, AuClaire, & Harris (1991)	—	—	44%[e]	9%[e]	—	—	n = 55 for treatment group; n = 58 for control group
Pearson, Masnyk, & King (1987)	90%	—	—	—	—	—	—
McDonald & Associates (1990); Yuan et al. (1990)	—	—	—	—	No significant differences between treatment and control groups[f]	—	N = 304; 152 families in treatment group; 152 families in control group
Feldman (1991)	92.7%	85.1%	54.2%	42.5%	—	—	n = 96 families in treatment group; n = 87 families in control group
Thieman & Dall (1992)	—	—	—	—	Statistically significant increase in family functioning from admission to termination	—	N = 995 families

Berry (1992)	96%	88%	94%[g]	—	N = 367 families
Leben & Smith (1992)	79%	62%[h]	—	—	N = 109 children
Henggeler, Melton, & Smith (1992)	—	—	58% (no rearrests)[i]	38% (no rearrests)[j]	N = 84 serious juvenile offenders; n = 43 in treatment group; n = 41 in control group
Henggeler et al. (1993)	—	—	39% (no rearrests)[i]	20% (no rearrests)[j]	N = 84 serious juvenile offenders; n = 43 in treatent group; n = 41 in control group
Henggeler, Schoenwald, Pickrel, et al. (1994), Missouri Delinquency Project	—	—	Families in the treatment group had more supportiveness, less conflict/hostility in family relations, and more cohesion and adapability. Adolescents in the treatment group had fewer behavior problems, and parents reported less symptomatology. For those who completed therapy, recidivism rates were 22% for the treatment group and 71% for the comparison group. Treatment group members were arrested less often and for less serious crimes.[k]	—	N = 200 chronic juvenile offenders

(continued)

Table 3.1. (continued)

	Percentage of children with family and other notable outcomes						Sample size
Authors	At service termination		At 12-month follow-up		At other frequencies of follow-up		
	Treatment	Control	Treatment	Control	Treatment	Control	
Henggeler, Schoenwald, Borduin, et al. (1994), Charleston, South Carolina	—	—	Treatment group had more gains in abstinence from substance abuse and delinquency and decreased institutionalization as compared with the control group.		—	—	n = 20 cases, adolescents with substance abuse and delinquency
Michigan Department of Social Services (1993)	—	—	24%	35%	7%/ 12%[g]	15%/ 26%[g]	N = 450 children; n = 225 in the treatment group; n = 225 in comparison group
Michigan Department of Social Services (1993)	—	—	19%	36%	5%/ 13%[g]	12%/ 26%[g]	N = 372 children (186 pairs) from previous sample referred due to abuse and/ or neglect only
Collier & Hill (1993)[m]	—	—	Treatment group had fewer recurrences of arrests, convictions, and incarcerations compared with the control group.		—	—	N = 80 families; n = 40 in treatment group; n = 40 in comparison group

Study							
Wells & Whittington (1993)	—	—	—			Functioning improved between admission and discharge; no decline between discharge and follow-up. Many problems apparent at admission were resolved or improved. Total of 59% remained in the home in which they lived at discharge.	N = 42 families

FAMILY REUNIFICATION SERVICES[n]

Study							
Walton et al., (1993)	93%	28.3%	75.4%	49%	70%	41.5%	n = 57 in treatment group; n = 53 in control group
Fein & Staff (1993)	—	—	—	—	38%[o] 28%[p]	—	N = 68 children
Woodworth, Hyde, Jordan, & Burchard (1994)	—	—	—	—	Restrictiveness of placements was less in the period after family preservation services than in the period prior to out-of-home state placement.[q]		N = 30 youth

[a] Participants were status-offending youth.
[b] WA, Washington State; UT, Utah.
[c] Average placement prevention rate was 93%; 92.9% represents only "official placements"; 92.3% represents all placements, including with relatives.
[d] This figure represents only "official placements."
[e] Cases were followed from 12 to 16 months, depending on when the case was selected. These figures represent only "official placement" rates; no significant difference was revealed when placement with relatives was considered.
[f] Follow-up at 8 months.
[g] Follow-up at 6 months.
[h] Follow-up data collected at end of 2-year project.
[i] Follow-up at 59 weeks postreferral.
[j] Follow-up at 120 weeks postreferral.
[k] Follow-up at 4 years.
[l] Follow-up at 3 years.
[m] Adjudicated juvenile deliquents.
[n] Rates of reunification for youth already in out-of-home placements.
[o] Family reunification rates *throughout* first 2 years.
[p] Family reunification rates *at end of* first 2 years.
[q] After receiving 6 months of family preservation services.

Although it appears that many family preservation programs have proven effective in keeping families intact and preventing or delaying the placement of children deemed at risk for substitute care, the effects do not appear to be long-lasting, and families continue to be at risk after service termination; it appears that treatment gains decrease as the amount of time after discharge increases. In an examination of factors related to successful adaptation after termination of services, Wells and Whittington (1993) found that child and family factors (risk of child removal at admission and formal and informal support of parent after discharge) were more strongly related to family functioning at follow-up than were treatment factors (engagement in treatment and resolution of admission problems at discharge). Furthermore, families with a child at imminent risk of removal at admission were found to be less likely to engage in treatment and less likely to have a high level of family health at follow-up than were those with children at lower risk for out-of-home placement.

In an appraisal of the major evaluations of family preservation programs, Rossi (1992) concluded that, although the majority of evaluations involved randomized experiments or close approximations of such designs, definitive findings concerning effectiveness cannot yet be ascertained. Small sample sizes and the use of overly simplified analysis strategies were also noted as common problem areas in evaluations included in the review. Furthermore, the majority of studies currently available have used a single-outcome criterion (i.e., rate of placement prevention). A number of evaluators have criticized the use of placement prevention rates as the single criterion to determine the effectiveness of family preservation services (Rossi, 1992). In fact, it has been argued that placement

> is an ambiguous indicator of treatment failure. Placement may be a positive outcome for some children. It may be affected by factors unrelated to the functioning of a family or a child, such as the availability of placement resources in a community. Moreover, research has shown that the majority of children admitted to intensive family preservation programs would *not* [italics added] have been placed without the program. Thus, it is difficult to use ab-

sence of placement as an indicator of success. (Wells & Whittington, 1993, p. 57)

In addition to placement prevention rates, research endeavors must include other criteria, such as the stability of the child's living situation, the quality of the child's living situation (Wells & Whittington, 1993), and changes in the well-being of the child and family (Rossi, 1992).

In addition to the concerns presented above, Usher (1993) asserts that many studies have found little or no difference in the effectiveness of family preservation services in decreasing out-of-home placement rates due to imprecise targeting of admission to family preservation programs and inconsistency in service delivery. He argues that evaluations were conducted despite awareness that these problematic issues were present. For example, evaluations of recently developed programs (Rossi, 1992) or those that are poorly managed are unlikely to reveal positive outcomes.

In light of these and other relevant issues, a number of recommendations for future research can be made. Certainly, definitive conclusions regarding the effectiveness of family preservation services await further research. Wells and Biegel (1991, 1992) have offered recommendations for future research in this area. These recommendations were based on the available research and discussions held at the 1989 National Conference on Intensive Family Preservation Services. Recommendations for future research included the following: 1) investigations to determine what portion of children approved for out-of-home placements meets the criteria to receive intensive home-based services; 2) outcome evaluations to determine the degree to which home-based services are meeting goals (i.e., the prevention of out-of-home placement and the reduction of future crises that may lead to placement); 3) longitudinal evaluations to assess the maintenance of treatment outcomes over time; 4) investigations to evaluate the impact of the ecological features of the program on implementation, functioning, and outcomes; 5) process evaluations to examine the clinical assumptions underlying treatment models and the ways in which clinicians and clients experience programs; 6) comprehensive evaluations of the functioning of children and their families at service termination; 7) investigations of service cost that take into account all services used by families during treatment and after termination; and 8) investigations to explore and examine those factors that act as facilitators and barriers to the replication of services across various settings. More recently, a reorientation for future research in the area of family preservation services has been proposed. Wells (1994) has suggested that research be placed in a theoretical framework; that research studies investigate critical outcomes, both intermediate and ultimate; and that research from related fields, such as foster care, be used to determine further areas for family preservation services research.

REFERENCES

Achenbach, T.M., & Edelbrock, C. (1983a). *Manual for the child behavior checklist and revised child behavior profile.* Burlington: University of Vermont, Department of Psychiatry.

Achenbach, T.M., & Edelbrock, C. (1983b). *Manual for the youth self-report and profile.* Burlington: University of Vermont, Department of Psychiatry.

Adoption Assistance and Child Welfare Act of 1980, PL 96-272. (June 17, 1980). Title 42, U.S.C. 1305 et seq: *U.S. Statutes at Large, 94,* 500–535.

Anders-Cibik, P., Zarski, J., Cleminshaw, H., & Greenbank, M. (1990, March). *Treating emotionally disturbed youth: Home-based family focused intervention.* Paper presented at the Annual Meeting of the American Association for Counseling and Development, Cincinnati, OH.

AuClaire, P., & Schwartz, I.M. (1986). *An evaluation of the effectiveness of intensive home-based services as an alternative to placement for adolescents and their families.* Minneapolis: University of Minnesota, Hubert H. Humphrey Institute of Public Affairs.

Berry, M. (1992). An evaluation of family preservation services: Fitting agency services to family needs. *Social Work, 37*(4), 314–321.

Burns, B., & Friedman, R.M. (1990). Examining the research base for child mental health services and policy. *Journal of Mental Health Administration, 17*(1), 87–98.

Child Welfare League of America. (1989). *Standards for services to strengthen and preserve families with children* (pp. 71–88). Washington, DC: Author.

Cole, E., & Duva, J. (1990). *Family preservation: An orientation for administrators & practitioners.* Washington, DC: Child Welfare League of America.

Collier, W.V., & Hill, R.H. (1993). *Family Ties intensive family preservation services program: An evaluation report.* New York: New York City Department of Juvenile Justice.

Epstein, N., Baldwin, L., & Bishop, D. (1983). The McMaster Family Assessment Device. *Journal of Marital and Family Therapy, 9,* 171–180.

Fein, E., & Staff, I. (1993). Last best chance: Findings from a reunification services program. *Child Welfare, 72*(1), 25–40.

Feldman, L.H. (1991). Evaluating the impact of intensive family preservation services in New Jersey. In K. Wells & D. Biegel (Eds.), *Family preservation services: Research and evaluation* (pp. 47–71). Newbury Park, CA: Sage Publications.

Forsythe, P. (1992). Homebuilders and family preservation. *Children and Youth Services Review, 14*, 37–47.

Fraser, M.W., Pecora, P.J., & Haapala, D.A. (1988). *Families in crisis: Final report on the family-based intensive treatment program.* Salt Lake City: University of Utah, Social Research Institute.

Haapala, D.A., & Kinney, J.M. (1988). Avoiding out-of-home placement of high-risk status offenders through the use of intensive home-based family preservation services. *Criminal Justice and Behavior, 15*(3), 334–348.

Hawkins, R., Almeida, M.C., Fabry, B., & Reitz, A.L. (1992). A scale to measure restrictiveness of living environments for troubled children and youths. *Hospital and Community Psychiatry, 43*, 54–58.

Henggeler, S.W., Melton, G.M., & Smith, L.A. (1992). Family preservation using multisystemic therapy: An effective alternative to incarcerating serious juvenile offenders. *Journal of Consulting and Clinical Psychology, 60*(6), 953–961.

Henggeler, S.W., Melton, G.M., Smith, L.A., Schoenwald, S.K., & Hanley, J.H. (1993). Family preservation using multisystemic treatment: Long-term follow-up to a clinical trial with serious juvenile offenders. *Journal of Child and Family Studies, 2*(4), 283–293.

Henggeler, S.W., Schoenwald, S.K., Borduin, C.M., Pickrel, S., Brondino, M.J., Rowland, M.D., & Scherer, D.G. (1994). Family preservation using multisystemic treatment with adolescent offenders and substance abusers: Long-term outcome, current projects, and interagency collaboration. In C.J. Liberton, K. Kutash, & R.M. Friedman (Eds.), *The 6th Annual Research Conference Proceedings, A System of Care for Children's Mental Health: Expanding the Research Base* (pp. 207–211). Tampa: University of South Florida, Florida Mental Health Institute, Research and Training Center for Children's Mental Health.

Henggeler, S.W., Schoenwald, S.K., Pickrel, S.G., Rowland, M.D., & Santos, A.B. (1994). The contribution of treatment outcome research to the reform of children's mental health services: Multisystemic therapy as an example. *Journal of Mental Health Administration, 21*(3), 229–239.

Hinckley, E.C., & Ellis, W.F. (1985). An effective alternative to residential placement: Home-based services. *Journal of Clinical Child Psychology, 14*(3), 209–213.

Hutchinson, J. (1982). *A comparative analysis of the costs of substitute care and family based services.* Iowa City: The University of Iowa School of Social Work, National Resource Center on Family Based Services.

Kinney, J., Haapala, D., & Booth, C. (1991). *Keeping families together: The Homebuilders model.* New York: Aldine DeGruyter.

Kinney, J., Madsen, B., Fleming, T., & Haapala, D. (1977). Homebuilders: Keeping families together. *Journal of Consulting and Clinical Psychology, 45*(4), 667–673.

Knitzer, J., & Yelton, S. (1990). Collaboration between child welfare and mental health: Both systems must exploit the program possibilities. *Public Welfare, 48*, 24–33.

Leben, C., & Smith, M.G. (1992). Reaching high-risk families and children: Results from two Texas intensive family intervention projects. In K. Kutash, C.J. Liberton, A. Algarin, & R.M. Friedman (Eds.), *The 5th Annual Research Conference Proceedings, A System of Care for Children's Mental Health: Expanding the Research Base* (pp. 207–215). Tampa: University of South Florida, Florida Mental Health Institute, Research and Training Center for Children's Mental Health.

Magura, S., Moses, B.S., & Jones, M.A. (1987). *Assessing risk and measuring change in families: The family risk scales.* Washington, DC: Child Welfare League of America.

McDonald & Associates, Inc. (1990). *Evaluation of AB1562 in-home care demonstration projects (Vol. 1: Final report).* Sacramento, CA: Author.

Michigan Department of Social Services. (1993). *Families First evaluation: Executive report.* Lansing, Michigan: University Associates.

National Resource Center on Family-Based Services. (1991). *Annotated directory of selected family-based programs.* Iowa City: University of Iowa, Oakdale Campus, School of Social Work.

New York City Department of Juvenile Justice. (1993). *Family Ties intensive family preservation services program: A financial analysis.* New York: Author.

Omnibus Budget Reconciliation Act of 1993, Family Preservation and Support Services, PL 103–66 (August 10, 1993). Title 42, U.S.C. 629 et seq: *U.S. Statutes at Large, 107,* 312–685.

Pearson, C.L., Masnyk, K., & King, P. (1987). *Intensive family services: Preliminary evaluation report.* Baltimore: Maryland Department of Human Resources.

Pecora, P.J., Fraser, M.W., & Haapala, D.A. (1991). Client outcomes and issues for program design. In K. Wells & D.E. Biegel (Eds.), *Family preservation services: Research and evaluation* (pp. 3–32). Newbury Park, CA: Sage Publications.

Pecora, P.J., Fraser, M.W., & Haapala, D.A. (1992). Intensive home-based family preservation services: An update from the FIT project. *Child Welfare, 71*(2), 177–188.

Polsky, D. (1986, April). Keeping the kids at home: Crisis intervention therapists help families stay together when the courts want to break them up. *Youth Policy,* pp. 21–23.

Rossi, P.H. (1992). Strategies for evaluation. *Children and Youth Services Review, 14*(1–2), 167–191.

Schwartz, I.M., AuClaire, P., & Harris, L.J. (1991). Family preservation services as an alternative to the out-of-home placement of adolescents: The Hennepin County experience. In K. Wells & D.E. Biegel (Eds.), *Family preservation services: Research and evaluation* (pp. 33–46). Newbury Park, CA: Sage Publications.

Stroul, B.A., & Goldman, S.K. (1990). Study of community-based services for children and adolescents who are severely emotionally disturbed. *Journal of Mental Health Administration, 17*(1), 61–77.

Thieman, A.A., & Dall, P.W. (1992). Family preservation services: Problems of measurement and assessment of risk. *Family Relations, 41*(2), 186–191.

Usher, L. (1993, October). *Balancing stakeholder interests in evaluations of innovative programs to serve families and children.* Paper presented at the annual meeting of the Association for Policy Analysis and Management, Washington, DC.

Walton, E., Fraser, M.W., Lewis, R.E., Pecora, P.J., & Walton, W.K. (1993). In-home family-focused reunification: An experimental study. *Child Welfare, 72*(5), 473–487.

Wells, K. (1994). A reorientation to knowledge development in family preservation services: A proposal. *Child Welfare, 73*(5), 475–488.

Wells, K., & Biegel, D.E. (1991). Conclusion. In K. Wells & D.E. Biegel (Eds.), *Family preservation services: Research and evaluation* (pp. 241–250). Newbury Park, CA: Sage Publications.

Wells, K., & Biegel, D.E. (1992). Intensive family preservation services research: Current status and future agenda. *Social Work Research and Abstracts, 28*(1), 21–27.

Wells, K., & Whittington, D. (1993). Child and family functioning after intensive family preservation services. *Social Service Review, 67*(1), 55–83.

Whittaker, J.K., & Tracy, E.M. (1990). Family preservation services and education for social work practice: Stimulus and response. In J.K. Whittaker, J. Kinney, E.M. Tracy, & C. Booth (Eds.), *Reaching high-risk families: Intensive family preservation in human services* (pp. 1–11). New York: Aldine DeGruyter.

Woodworth, K., Hyde, K., Jordan, K., & Burchard, J. (1994, February). *"Wrapping" services in an urban setting: Outcomes of urban service reform.* Paper presented at The 7th Annual Research Conference, A System of Care for Children's Mental Health: Expanding the Research Base, Tampa, FL.

Yelton, S. (1991). Family preservation from a mental health perspective. *The Child, Youth, and Family Services Quarterly, 14*(3), 6–8.

Yuan, Y.Y.T., McDonald, W.R., Wheeler, C.E., Struckman-Johnson, D., & Rivest, M. (1990). *Evaluation of AB 1562 in-home care demonstration projects. Volumes I and II.* Sacramento, CA: W.R. McDonald and Associates, Inc.

CHAPTER 4

Therapeutic Foster Care

According to the Select Committee on Children, Youth, and Families (1990), an estimated 500,000 children were in out-of-home settings in the late 1980s, with an approximate increase to 840,000 expected by 1995. One of the most widely utilized forms of out-of-home placement for children with serious emotional disorders is therapeutic foster care (TFC), considered to be the least restrictive form of care among the range of residential services available to children with serious emotional disturbances (Stroul, 1989). In a review of the literature on specialized foster care programs, Webb (1988) found that nearly two thirds of the programs described their populations as children and adolescents with emotional or behavioral disturbances.

Therapeutic foster care is a relatively new form of treatment, with a variety of models having been developed across the country since the mid-1980s. This service approach has been defined broadly as

> a service which provides treatment for troubled children within the private homes of trained families. The approach combines the normalizing influence of family-based care with specialized treatment interventions, thereby creating a therapeutic environment in the context of a nurturant family home. (Stroul, 1989, p. 13)

A variety of terms have been used to describe therapeutic foster care, such as specialized foster family care, special foster care, treatment foster care, foster family-based treatment, individualized residential treatment, professional parenting, and intensive foster care. For the purposes of this review, the generic term *therapeutic foster care* will be used.

Although there is great variability among models and a lack of agreement regarding terminology, most TFC programs share common features. These general characteristics include the following: Children are placed with foster parents who have been carefully selected to work with children with

69

special needs; foster parents receive preservice and/or in-service education or training to assist them in working effectively with the child; with occasional exceptions, only one child is placed in a home at a time; program staff have small caseloads, which allows them to work closely and intensively with each child and family; a support system is developed among foster care parents; foster parents receive a special stipend that is significantly higher than the rate provided to traditional foster parents; and biological families are provided with counseling, support, and other types of assistance (Meadowcroft, 1989; Stroul, 1989). TFC programs differ in such areas as treatment approach, structure, intensity, type of training and support provided, and amount of payment to foster care parents (Research and Training Center for Children's Mental Health, 1986).

A number of advantages of therapeutic foster care programs over other residential services have been noted in the literature. One advantage is the flexibility of the programs. It is possible to provide services to children of varying ages and with a variety of presenting problems. Furthermore, TFC provides a less restrictive and more natural environment for treatment; the generalization of treatment gains is enhanced because of the family environment; TFC services are highly individualized; children receive a sense of "connectedness"; and TFC is viewed more positively than other residential treatment programs. With regard to cost, therapeutic foster care programs are relatively easy and inexpensive to start. This is attributed primarily to the fact that no special facility is needed, and programs can be started on a small scale with only a few staff and a limited number of treatment homes. Additionally, the cost of therapeutic foster care is lower in comparison with other residential placement settings (Stroul, 1989; Stroul & Friedman, 1986).

COST COMPARISONS AND COST SAVINGS

Therapeutic foster care programs are typically the least expensive service in the range of residential services available to children with serious emotional disturbances (Stroul & Friedman, 1986). Because of the wide disparity among payments made to treatment parents and disparity in methods of cost calculation, the reported costs of TFC vary significantly. An overview of the costs of various TFC programs, which range from $35 per day to $150 per day, has been provided (see Stroul, 1989).

Despite this wide variation in cost, TFC compares favorably with the cost of other residential services. A survey conducted by Snodgrass and Bryant (1989) revealed that over 90% of the TFC programs reported costs to be lower than costs for group homes or institutional placement settings. Other studies and reviews have documented similar cost savings.

Bryant (1981) provided evidence of the cost savings of early therapeutic foster care programs. For example, the Alberta Parent Counselors Program provided therapeutic foster care services to children with emotional disturbances at half the cost of residential care, and the Massachusetts Treatment Alternative Project served children who were scheduled to enter a residential placement setting at two thirds the cost. People Places provided treatment to children with serious disturbances at half the cost of institutional placement.

A comparison of the costs of TFC and other residential treatment settings in California was conducted by Beggs (1987). Again, TFC was estimated to cost less than group homes, subacute facilities, and acute hospitals. Hawkins, Almeida, and Samet (1990) conducted a comparison study of a foster family–based treatment program (PRYDE) and five other out-of-home placement choices (residential treatment centers, specialized foster care settings, group homes, intensive treatment units, and parents). Results revealed that placement in the PRYDE program was less expensive, on a daily basis, than the other placement choices included in the study, with the exception of specialized foster care.

Chamberlain and Reid (1991) examined the cost of a specialized foster care program for youth who had been previously hospitalized. At the time of the study, the hospital program cost was $6,000 per month, whereas the cost for the experimental program (specialized foster care) was $3,000 per month. Placement in the specialized foster care program saved an average of $10,280 per case in hospitalization costs.

The Kaleidoscope program also reported substantial cost savings with regard to their Therapeutic Foster Family Program (Kaleidoscope, Inc., n.d.). Cost of treatment in a state institution was estimated to be about $40,000 per child per year, whereas the cost of the Individualized Treatment Program of Kaleidoscope was $72 per child per day (or $26,280 annually).

The cost of the Mentor Program (Mikkelsen, Bereika, & McKenzie, 1993) was considerably less, in comparison with inpatient hospitalization. The average cost per admission to the Mentor Program was reported as $3,825, whereas the cost per admission for psychiatric hospitalization was $18,030.

EFFECTIVENESS AND OUTCOME RESEARCH

As a means of evaluating the effectiveness of a TFC program, most studies have examined discharge data. Successful discharge is defined as a situation in which the child leaves the TFC program and enters a less restrictive setting (e.g., biological home, adoptive home, foster home, or independent living situation). Stroul (1989) presented a review of discharge data for a number of therapeutic foster home programs. Overall, the data indicated that successful discharge rates ranged from a low of 62% to a high of 89%. A more recent survey of treatment family-based foster care programs in the United States and Canada conducted by Galaway, Nutter, and Hudson (1995) revealed that 63% of the children discharged from these programs were placed in less restrictive settings.

Although many excellent therapeutic foster care programs have been established to meet the needs of children and families, most of the available literature consists primarily of program descriptions, with few attempts to examine effectiveness (Burns & Friedman, 1990; Galaway et al., 1995; Webb, 1988; Woolf, 1990). Despite the paucity of research, a review of the available literature, published and unpublished, on the effectiveness of TFC is presented in the following sections. For an overview of descriptive studies of the program characteristics of therapeutic foster care, see Meadowcroft, Thomlison, and Chamberlain (1994).

People Places

People Places, which began operating in Virginia in 1973, represents one of the first therapeutic foster care programs established for children with serious emotional disorders (Bryant & Snodgrass, 1992). For 1977, Witters and Snodgrass (cited in Stroul, 1989) reported that, of all admissions ($N = 26$), 89% were discharged to less restrictive settings, whereas the remaining 11% were placed in institutions. Discharge data from 1981 revealed that, of the children admitted ($N = 45$), 86% were discharged to less restrictive settings (Jones, 1990). Improvements in child functioning on various target behaviors from time of admission to discharge were assessed also. For the two samples mentioned above, greater than 75% of the target behaviors were rated by staff as significantly improved. Target behaviors were rated again at 2 months ($n = 26$) and 7 months ($n = 25$) postdischarge. An average of 80% of the target behaviors were considered to be "no problem" or "some problem, but improving" (Jones, 1990; Snodgrass & Campbell, 1981). Discharge data were collected for the 50 youth discharged from People Places during the 3-year period of 1989–1991 (Bryant & Snodgrass, 1992). The majority (79%) were discharged to a less restrictive setting. Furthermore, 68% had attained their permanency planning goal of adoption or return to family or relatives.

Professional Parenting
The Professional Parenting program was developed in 1979 by the Bringing It All Back Home (BIABH) Study Center in North Carolina. This program represents a less intensive and less structured model of TFC in that the treatment program is relatively unstructured and relies on the therapeutic value of the home environment and the skills of the treatment foster parents. More structured and intensive treatment services are provided if the initial program appears inadequate. Jones (1990) reported that, of the 24 children discharged, 79% of the children were in less restrictive placements upon discharge. The remaining 21% were placed in more restrictive settings, such as psychiatric hospitals, detention centers, or training schools.

Pressley Ridge Youth Development Extension (PRYDE)

Pressley Ridge Youth Development Extension (PRYDE), established in 1981, is a highly structured and intensive foster family–based treatment program for children and adolescents identified as troubled. The main feature of the PRYDE model is the philosophy of the "professional" parent as the primary "agent of treatment" rather than as a caregiver only. During 1984 (as of September), 13 of the 16 children in the PRYDE program had successful discharges. Thus, 82% of the youth had returned to a less restrictive setting within their community following discharge (Hawkins, Meadowcroft, Trout, & Luster, 1985). Discharge data from 1981–1987 revealed that 72% of the children ($N = 114$) had been placed in less restrictive settings upon discharge. In terms of long-term postdischarge status, 73% remained in less restrictive settings 1–2 years after discharge (Jones, 1990).

Follow-up data on all children discharged from a PRYDE program were gathered by phone annually. Follow-up data at 1 year for 86% of the 110 children discharged between July 1983 and June 1987 revealed that 76% of these children were living in less restrictive settings 1 year after discharge from the treatment home. A total of 77% were either in school or employed (Jones, 1990).

Hawkins et al. (1990) reported the preliminary findings of a comparative evaluation of the PRYDE program and five other out-of-home placement choices. Data were gathered from the files ($N = 461$) of the referring child welfare agency. A total of 26 children were served in PRYDE homes, and the remaining were placed in one of the other out-of-home settings. Again, the primary variable of interest was discharge status. On average, children discharged from the PRYDE program were more likely to be placed in less restrictive settings than were those in the other five placement settings. Furthermore, statistically significant differences were found between the level of restrictiveness for those discharged from PRYDE and those from residential treatment centers and intensive treatment units, as measured by the level of restrictiveness scale developed by the authors. The average level of restrictiveness of subsequent placements following discharge also was calculated. Children discharged from the PRYDE program tended to have equally or less restrictive subsequent placements than did children discharged from the other five placement settings. However, no data were collected on the level of restrictiveness prior to entering the PRYDE program; thus, it is not known if the children were comparable at admission.

Kaleidoscope, Inc.

Kaleidoscope, Inc. is a licensed, not-for-profit child welfare agency that strives to serve the most challenging children in the state of Illinois (Kaleidoscope, Inc., n.d.). One program component within Kaleidoscope is the Therapeutic Foster Family Homes Program. This program provides family living and specialized services on a daily basis to about 65 children and youth who would otherwise be placed in institutions. According to Stroul (1989), discharge data indicated that 62% of the children and youth served by this program were discharged to a less restrictive setting.

Oregon Social Learning Center: Transitions and Monitor

Studies were conducted to evaluate the effectiveness of two specialized foster care programs located at the Oregon Social Learning Center (Chamberlain & Reid, 1991; Chamberlain & Weinrott, 1990). *Transitions* is a specialized foster care program for children and youth with serious emotional disturbances; *Monitor* is a specialized foster care program for chronically delinquent youth.

An evaluation of the Transitions program utilized a randomized design in which children from the state hospital were assigned to the specialized foster care program ($n = 10$) or to other available treatment settings within their communities ($n = 10$). Children receiving specialized foster care services spent an average of 79% of their next year in family-based settings, whereas those in the comparison group spent only 49% of their time in the community. For the year after placement, the amount of time that children were maintained in community settings was compared for the experimental and control groups. The mean number of days living in community placements was not reliably different for the two groups. However, not all children in the control group ($n =$

7) actually received a placement outside of the hospital setting; therefore, the treatment condition appeared to serve as a mechanism for community placement for children with serious emotional disorders participating in this study.

In addition to an examination of discharge status, all participants in the study were assessed across a number of measures. Results of the Child Global Assessment Scale (CGAS) (Shaffer et al., 1983), used to measure level of functioning during the past month, indicated that children in both groups experienced major impairment in functioning in several areas. The Parent Daily Report Checklist (PDR) (Chamberlain & Reid, 1987), which measured the occurrence of problem behaviors during the previous 24-hour period, was administered at baseline, 3 months, and 7 months. A mean daily rate was calculated for the number of problem behaviors reported for each child at each of the three points in time. At baseline, both groups showed mean daily rates of over 20 reported problems per day. At 3 months, a decrease of over 50% was evident for those in the experimental group, whereas the control group showed no reduction in mean daily rate of problem behavior. At 7 months, the mean daily rate had decreased for the control group, but not to the level of the experimental group. Although a more rapid reduction in daily problem behaviors was evident for the experimental group, no significant group-by-time interaction effect was apparent.

The Behavior Symptom Inventory (BSI) (Derogatis & Spencer, 1982), a self-report inventory in which children rate their own level of functioning, was administered prior to placement and at 7 months after placement. Members of the experimental group reported twice as many problems as did those in the control group at both measurement points. The Adolescent Problem Inventory (API) (Gaffney & McFall, 1981), designed for youth 12 years and older, and the Taxonomy of Problematic Social Situations (TOPS) (Dodge, McClaskey, & Feldman, 1985), designed for children below the age of 12, were administered to assess the children's level of social competency. No significant improvement was observed for either group on these measures.

An evaluation was conducted to determine the effectiveness of the Monitor program, which provided specialized foster care services to 12- to 18-year-old youths who had a history of chronic delinquency (Chamberlain, 1990; Chamberlain & Weinrott, 1990). Youth ($N = 32$; 16 matched cases) in the Monitor program were matched to other youth who had similar characteristics and histories and who had been committed and diverted to traditional community treatment programs, such as group homes, residential treatment centers, or intensive probation. Data were gathered on the number of days incarcerated in state training schools during the 1-year follow-up period prior to placement in a diversion program, number of days in treatment, and number of days incarcerated during the 2-year postdischarge period. No significant differences were found for the two groups on number of days incarcerated during the pretreatment period or average amount of days in treatment. However, a greater number of youth in the Monitor group were incarcerated less frequently and for shorter periods of time than were those who received an alternative type of service. Furthermore, a greater proportion of youth in the Monitor program (75%) completed their community programs, in comparison with those in the control group (31%).

Follow-up data on institutionalization rates were gathered at 2 years for the two groups. Over the follow-up period, a significant difference was found between the groups. Of the youth in the experimental group, 50% were reincarcerated at least once during the follow-up period, compared with 94% of those receiving traditional services. Furthermore, a significant negative correlation was revealed between number of days in treatment and number of days of subsequent incarceration for those in the experimental group. No significant correlation was observed for those in the comparison group.

The Mentor Program
The Mentor Program, a short-term, family-based residential treatment model, was developed to serve as an alternative to psychiatric hospitalization for children (Mikkelsen et al., 1993). The program utilized a multidisciplinary team of professionals and mentors (specially trained individuals) who

worked with the child and the biological family within the home of the mentor. The program shares a number of similarities with treatment foster care; however, differences are evident. The principal difference between treatment foster care and the Mentor Program is the function of the program, because the Mentor Program is designed to provide acute care on a more short-term basis.

Outcome data for 112 consecutive admissions revealed that, at discharge, 72% of the children with planned discharges were returned to their family or relatives, 17% were placed in long-term specialized foster care settings, 5% were placed in group homes, and 6% were placed in psychiatric hospitals or residential treatment centers. Follow-up data at 3 months ($N = 61$ discharged children) indicated that 67% were living at home or with relatives; 12% were in foster care placements; 5% were in specialized foster care settings; 11% were in residential placements such as hospitals, residential treatment centers, or substance abuse treatment facilities; and 5% were categorized as "other" or "unspecified."

Maryland Department of Human Resources

The Maryland Department of Human Resources (1987) examined the effectiveness of specialized foster care services by evaluating improvement in functioning at time of placement and 6 months after discharge. Measures of functioning revealed that almost all categories of behavior problems decreased for children receiving therapeutic foster care services, whereas behavior problems increased for those in the control group.

San Francisco Bay Programs

In a report of therapeutic foster care programs in the San Francisco Bay area, Beggs (1987) presented the following discharge data for three programs. Future Families, in Aptos, California, reported that 78% of youth in the program were discharged to less restrictive settings, whereas 18% were placed in residential treatment settings. The San Francisco Therapeutic Family Homes Program reported that 80% of youth in the program were discharged to less restrictive settings, whereas 17% were placed in residential treatment centers. The St. Vincent's School for Boys, in San Rafael, California, reported that only 13% were discharged to more restrictive settings, such as residential treatment or group homes.

Missouri Division of Family Services
Bryant, Simmens, and McKee (1989) reported discharge data for the Missouri Division of Family Services Foster Family Treatment Program. Data indicated that 74% of youth in the program were placed in less restrictive settings upon discharge from the program.

Programs in England
Two studies examining specialist foster family care practices in England have provided support for their effectiveness. Practices were based on the Swedish model of community care for adolescents, which incorporates the principles of normalization, localization, voluntariness, and participation. An examination of the Kent Family Placement Project (Hazel, 1989) revealed that the program was effective in serving as an alternative to residential or custodial care for adolescents identified as delinquent or severely troubled. In a comparison of specialist foster family care practices and residential child care practices, Colton (1990) found that, overall, the specialist foster family care programs were significantly more child oriented than the residential placement settings on four dimensions of care: management of daily events; children's involvement in community activities; provision of physical amenities; and controls and sanctions used by caregivers.

CONCLUSIONS AND FUTURE RESEARCH NEEDS
Therapeutic foster care is a relatively recent form of care for children and youth with serious emotional problems and has become one of the most widely used forms of treatment for this population. There is wide variability among the models of TFC that have been developed and implemented across the United States and in England. TFC programs may differ along the dimensions of treatment approach; structure and intensity; and type of training, support, and stipend provided to treatment foster care parents; but they do share some com-

monalities. As a result of this wide variability, conclusions and generalizations regarding the effectiveness of therapeutic foster care are difficult to reach.

In an examination of the available research on children's mental health services, Burns and Friedman (1990) reported the results of only two studies of TFC effectiveness. A number of additional studies have been conducted since that review; however, there are few that truly investigate effectiveness by using comparison groups. The studies and evaluations of TFC programs included in the current review revealed successful discharge rates ranging from 62% to 89%; that is, between 62% and 89% of the children who received therapeutic foster care services were placed in less restrictive settings upon discharge (see Table 4.1). This result is similar to the range reported by Stroul (1989) in her review of TFC programs. A 1995 survey of treatment family-based foster care programs in the United States and Canada revealed that 63% of the children are discharged to less restrictive settings (Galaway et al., 1995).

Although the majority of studies have examined discharge rates as the single-outcome criterion, a few studies have investigated the effects of therapeutic foster care services on child functioning (Chamberlain & Reid, 1991; Chamberlain & Weinrott, 1990; Jones, 1990; Maryland Department of Human Resources, 1987), time spent in family-based settings (Chamberlain & Reid, 1991; Chamberlain & Weinrott, 1990), and rates of incarceration and arrests (Chamberlain, 1990; Chamberlain & Weinrott, 1990). In general, these studies have reported favorable outcomes for TFC on these dimensions. The data seem to suggest that TFC services have the potential to effectively serve a number of children who would otherwise be treated in more restrictive placement settings and can have a positive impact on functioning, adjustment, delinquency, time spent in family-based settings, and other outcomes. Furthermore, cost savings associated with TFC in comparison with other residential treatment settings have been documented. However, only two of the studies reviewed in this chapter used a controlled design to examine the effectiveness of TFC in comparison with other forms of treatment. The results from these studies were mixed; the re-

Table 4.1. Effectiveness of therapeutic foster care programs: Discharge status rates and other outcomes

Program and authors	Percentage of children in less restrictive setting at time of discharge		Percentage of children in less restrictive settings at time of follow-up		Sample size
	Treatment group	Control group	Treatment group	Control group	
PRYDE: Hawkins, Meadowcroft, Trout, & Luster (1985)	82%	—	—	—	N = 16
PRYDE: Jones (1990)[a]	72%	—	—	—	N = 114
PRYDE: Jones (1990)	—	—	73%[b]	—	—
PRYDE: Hawkins, Almeida, & Samet (1990)	On average, children from PRYDE experienced less restrictive placements than did children from 5 other settings.	—	—	—	N = 461
PRYDE: Jones (1990)	—	—	76%[c]	—	N = 95
People Places: Jones (1990); Stroul (1989)	1977: 89% 1981: 86% For both samples, >75% of target behaviors improved.	—	At follow-up 80% of target problem behaviors were improving or were no longer a problem.[d]	—	N = 26 (1977) N = 45 (1981)
People Places: Bryant & Snodgrass (1992)	79%	—	—	—	N = 50

(continued)

Table 4.1. (continued)

Program and authors	Percentage of children in less restrictive setting at time of discharge		Percentage of children in less restrictive settings at time of follow-up		Sample size
	Treatment group	Control group	Treatment group	Control group	
Professional Parenting: Jones (1990)	79.2%	—	—	—	N = 24
Kaleidoscope: Stroul (1989)	62%	—	—	—	N = 65
Transitions Program (Oregon Social Learning Center): Chamberlain & Reid (1991); Chamberlain & Weinrott (1990)[e]	Children spent an average of 79% of their next year in family-based settings.	Children spent an average of 49% in the community; only 40% were in family-based placements.	Decrease in problem behavior occurred.[f] No improvement in level of social competency occurred.	Decrease in problem behavior occurred, but did not reach level of treatment group.[g] No improvement in level of social competency occurred.	N = 20 (n = 10 in treatment group; n = 10 in control group)
Monitor program (Oregon Social Learning Center): Chamberlain (1990); Chamberlain & Weinrott (1990)	Youth in the treatment group were incarcerated less frequently and for shorter periods of time. 75% completed community program.	31% completed program.	50% were incarcerated at least once.[h]	94% were incarcerated at least once.[h]	N = 32 (16 matched cases)
The Mentor Program: Mikkelsen, Bereika, & McKenzie (1993)	72% were released to family or relatives, 17% to TFC settings.	—	67% were released to family or relatives, 5% in TFC settings, 12% in foster care.	—	N = 112 (at discharge) N = 61 (at follow-up)

			Almost all areas of problem behaviors decreased.	Behavior problems increased.
Maryland Department of Human Resources (1987)	—	—		Behavior problems increased.
Future Families: Beggs (1987)	78%	—	—	
San Francisco Therapeutic Family Homes Program: Beggs (1987)	80%	—	—	
St. Vincent's School for Boys: Beggs (1987)	87%	—	—	
Missouri Division of Family Services Foster Family Treatment Program: Bryant, Simmens, & McKee (1989)	74%	—	—	

Note: Therapeutic foster care (TFC), service approach that provides treatment to children within private homes of trained families (also called specialized foster family care, treatment foster care, intensive foster care). Discharge status rates, percentage of children receiving "successful discharge"—when child is able to go to less restrictive setting.

[a]Discharge data from 1981–1987.
[b]1–2 years after discharge.
[c]1-year data for those discharged 1983–1987.
[d]At 2 months and 7 months postdischarge.
[e]Data for December 1989–December 1991.
[f]At 3-month follow-up.
[g]At 7-month follow-up.
[h]At 2-year follow-up.

sults of one study showed no differences in community tenure at follow-up, whereas the other found significantly lower rates of incarceration and length of time incarcerated, both during treatment as well as during the follow-up period, for youth enrolled in TFC programs. Although these studies provide a start in examining the effectiveness of TFC as compared with other forms of treatment, both were based on small samples of children and point to the need for further investigations using controlled designs to fully investigate the effectiveness of TFC.

Several other directions for future research have been noted in the literature (see Friedman, 1989; Meadowcroft et al., 1994). Most evaluations have pointed to the general effectiveness of TFC; however, more specific issues must be addressed, such as determining which populations of children and youth are best served by TFC. Research must continue to compare TFC with other institutional treatment alternatives, as well as with nonresidential placement options. In addition to child functioning, research must investigate the impact of TFC on socially significant areas of children's lives, such as school attendance, employment, or protection from harm. Evaluations must focus on determining the critical variables (child, family, and service) that are necessary to produce successful outcomes and to develop empirically based guidelines. Finally, efforts must be undertaken to examine the long-term effects of TFC for children and their families.

REFERENCES

Beggs, M. (1987). *Foster families as partners in therapy: Four therapeutic foster care programs in the Bay Area*. San Francisco, CA: San Francisco Study Center, Zellerbach Family Fund.

Bryant, B. (1981). Special foster care: A history and rationale. *Journal of Clinical Child Psychology, 10*(1), 8–20.

Bryant, B., Simmens, F., & McKee, M. (1989). Doing it in public: A review of foster family treatment program development in Missouri. In J. Hudson & B. Galaway (Eds.), *Specialist foster family care: A normalizing experience* (pp. 159–175). New York: Haworth Press.

Bryant, B., & Snodgrass, R.D. (1992). Foster family care applications with special populations: People Places, Inc. *Community Alternatives: International Journal of Family Care, 4*(2), 1–25.

Burns, B.J., & Friedman, R.M. (1990). Examining the research base for child mental health services and policy. *Journal of Mental Health Administration, 17*(1), 87–98.

Chamberlain, P. (1990). Comparative evaluation of specialized foster care for seriously delinquent youths: A first step. *Community Alternatives: International Journal of Family Care, 2*(2), 21–36.

Chamberlain, P., & Reid, J.B. (1987). Parent observation and report of child symptoms. *Behavioral Assessment, 9,* 97–109.

Chamberlain, P., & Reid, J.B. (1991). Using a specialized foster care community treatment model for children and adolescents leaving the state mental hospital. *Journal of Community Psychology, 19*(3), 266–276.

Chamberlain, P., & Weinrott, M. (1990). Specialized foster care: Treating seriously emotionally disturbed children. *Children Today, 19*(1), 24–27.

Colton, M. (1990). Specialist foster family and residential child care practices. *Community Alternatives: International Journal of Family Care, 2*(2), 1–20.

Derogatis, L.R., & Spencer, P.M. (1982). *The Brief Symptom Inventory (BSI) administration, scoring, & procedures manual–I.* Baltimore: Clinical Psychometric Research.

Dodge, K.A., McClaskey, C.L., & Feldman, E.L. (1985). A situational approach to the assessment of social competence in children. *Journal of Consulting and Clinical Psychology, 53,* 344–353.

Friedman, R.M. (1989). The role of therapeutic foster care in an overall system of care: Issues in service delivery and program evaluation. In R.P. Hawkins & J. Breiling (Eds.), *Therapeutic foster care: Critical issues* (pp. 205–219). Washington, DC: Child Welfare League of America.

Gaffney, L.R., & McFall, R.M. (1981). A comparison of social skills in delinquent and nondelinquent adolescent girls using a behavioral role–playing inventory. *Journal of Consulting and Clinical Psychology, 49,* 959–967.

Galaway, B., Nutter, R.W., & Hudson, J. (1995). Relationship between discharge outcomes for treatment foster-care clients and program characteristics. *Journal of Emotional and Behavioral Disorders, 3*(1), 46–54.

Hawkins, R.P., Almeida, M.C., & Samet, M. (1990). Comparative evaluation of foster-family-based treatment and five other placement choices: A preliminary report. In A. Algarin, R.M. Friedman, A.J. Duchnowski, K. Kutash, S. Silver, & M.K. Johnson (Eds.), *The 2nd Annual Conference Proceedings on Children's Mental Health Services and Policy: Building a Research Base* (pp. 91–111). Tampa: University of South Florida, Florida Mental Health Institute, Research and Training Center for Children's Mental Health.

Hawkins, R.P., Meadowcroft, P., Trout, B.A., & Luster, W.C. (1985). Foster family–based treatment. *Journal of Clinical Child Psychology, 14*(3), 220–228.

Hazel, N. (1989). Adolescent fostering as a community resource. *Community Alternatives: International Journal of Family Care, 1*(1), 1–10.

Jones, R.J. (1990). Evaluating therapeutic foster care. In P. Meadowcroft & B.A. Trout (Eds.), *Troubled youth in treatment homes: A handbook of therapeutic foster care* (pp. 143–181). Washington, DC: Child Welfare League of America.

Kaleidoscope, Inc. (n.d.). *Program materials.* Chicago, IL: Author.

Maryland Department of Human Resources. (1987). *Specialized foster care.* Baltimore: Department of Fiscal Services.

Meadowcroft, P. (1989). Treating emotionally disturbed children and adolescents in foster homes. In J. Hudson & B. Galaway (Eds.), *Specialist foster family care: A normalizing experience.* New York: Haworth Press.

Meadowcroft, P., Thomlison, B., & Chamberlain, P. (1994). Treatment foster care services: A research agenda for child welfare. *Journal of Child Welfare, 73*(5), 565–581.

Mikkelsen, E.J., Bereika, G.M., & McKenzie, J.C. (1993). Short–term family–based residential treatment: An alternative to psychiatric hospitalization for children. *American Journal of Orthopsychiatry, 63*(1), 28–33.

Research and Training Center for Children's Mental Health, Florida Mental Health Institute. (1986). Therapeutic foster care. *Update, 2*(1), 8–10.

Select Committee on Children, Youth, and Families, U.S. House of Representatives. (1990). *No place to call home: Discarded children in America* (HR #101-395). Washington, DC: Author.

Shaffer, D., Gould, M.S., Brasic, J., Ambrosini, P., Fisher, P., Bird, H., & Aluwahlia, S. (1983). A Children's Global Assessment Scale (CGAS). *Archives of General Psychiatry, 40*, 1228–1231.

Snodgrass, R., & Bryant, B. (1989). Special foster care and foster family-based treatment: A national program survey. In R.P. Hawkins & J. Breiling (Eds.), *Therapeutic foster care: Critical issues.* Washington, DC: Child Welfare League of America.

Snodgrass, R., & Campbell, R. (1981). *Specialized foster care: A community alternative to institutional placement.* Staunton, VA: People Places.

Stroul, B.A. (1989). *Series on community–based services for children and adolescents who are severely emotionally disturbed: Volume III: Therapeutic foster care.* Washington, DC: Georgetown University Child Development Center, National Technical Assistance Center for Children's Mental Health.

Stroul, B.A., & Friedman, R.M. (1986). *A system of care for children and youth with severe emotional disturbances* (rev. ed.). Washington, DC: Georgetown University Child Development Center, National Technical Assistance Center for Children's Mental Health.

Webb, D.B. (1988). Specialized foster care as an alternative therapeutic out-of-home placement model. *Journal of Clinical Child Psychology, 17*(1), 34–43.

Woolf, G.D. (1990). An outlook on foster care in the United States. *Child Welfare, 69*(1), 75–81.

CHAPTER 5

Crisis and Emergency Services

Within the system of care model proposed by Stroul and Friedman (1986), crisis and emergency services are defined as

> an important set of services that serve both youngsters who are basically well-functioning but experience periodic crises, and youngsters with longer-term, more serious problems who are prone to acute episodes at which time they require special services. (p. 51)

The underlying goal of crisis services is to assist the child and family in resolving the crisis situation and to avoid hospitalization.

Crisis and emergency services range from nonresidential to residential settings and involve various types of agencies, services, and personnel (Stroul & Goldman, 1990). Nonresidential crisis services include crisis prevention, identification, and management services; crisis telephone lines; emergency outpatient services; mobile crisis outreach services, including emergency medical teams; and intensive home-based interventions. In some cases, however, the needs of a child or family in crisis *cannot* be met adequately through nonresidential crisis services and require residential crisis services. Examples of residential crisis services include runaway shelters, crisis group homes, therapeutic foster care programs used for short-term crisis placements, hospital emergency rooms, and crisis stabilization units. When other approaches to crisis intervention are not appropriate, inpatient hospitalization serves as another source of temporary placement.

Despite this variability, community-based crisis services share a number of common characteristics. These characteristics, as outlined by Goldman (1988), are as follows:

1. Crisis services are available 24 hours a day, 7 days a week.

2. Community-based crisis programs share the common purpose of the prevention of hospitalization and the stabilization of the crisis situation in the most normalized setting available.
3. Crisis services are offered on a short-term basis.
4. The capacity of crisis programs tends to be limited to small numbers of youth.
5. Typically, crisis services include evaluation and assessment, crisis intervention and stabilization, and follow-up planning.
6. To the extent possible, families are involved in all phases of crisis treatment.
7. Staff in crisis programs tend to share similar characteristics, such as flexibility and adaptability, a high level of skill and competence, a high level of energy and dedication, an ability to establish a relationship quickly and to terminate, and the ability to work as part of a team.
8. Crisis programs usually are part of a larger agency that offers other services, such as inpatient, day treatment, or outpatient services.

FUNDING AND COST COMPARISONS

Information regarding the costs and financing of crisis and emergency programs for children is scarce. In a study of community-based services for children and adolescents with serious emotional disorders, Stroul and Goldman (1990) gathered financial data from a small number of crisis programs. Findings revealed that most programs were funded through a combination of sources that included contracts or funding support from state or local public sector human service agencies, federal grants, private sector funds, philanthropic donations, third-party reimbursements, and patient fees. Data on costs also were limited. Although costs were calculated in a variety of ways, making comparisons difficult, it was concluded that the costs of crisis programs "are dramatically less than the average cost of private psychiatric hospitals" (p. 73).

Few investigations of the cost savings associated with crisis programs have been conducted. Of those studies included in the present review, only four reported cost data.

The costs of the Children's Mobile Outreach Program (Moore, 1991) compared favorably with those associated with institutional programs, and the Systematic Crisis Intervention Program (Gutstein, Rudd, Graham, & Rayha, 1988) was found to be lower in cost compared with psychiatric hospitalization in the Houston area. Bishop and McNally (1993) reported that the cost of an in-home crisis intervention program in Buffalo, New York, resulted in a total savings of over $300,000 in hospital costs. Schweitzer and Dubey (1994) reported that a scattered-site crisis bed program in Suffolk County, New York, operated at about 10% of the cost of hospitalization. The average cost per day for a crisis bed placement was $74, whereas the cost was $678 per day for hospitalization in the state children's psychiatric center and up to $1,000 per day in a local private hospital. Due to the small number of evaluations that have included a cost comparison component, it is difficult to draw conclusions regarding the cost savings associated with crisis services.

EFFECTIVENESS AND OUTCOME RESEARCH

Adolescent Crisis Team and Respite House

Goldman (1988) provided an extensive overview of the Adolescent Crisis Team and Respite House, which operated from the South Shore Mental Health Center in Quincy, Massachusetts. The overarching goal of both programs was the provision of services to youth and their families who were experiencing serious behavioral, psychiatric, or emotional distress. The Adolescent Crisis Team was a multidisciplinary team of professionals that provided 24-hour emergency service to adolescents who were experiencing a crisis and to their families. The Respite House, a home located in a residential neighborhood, served as an alternative to psychiatric hospitalization for youth who were experiencing psychiatric crisis and were at risk of hospitalization. Services provided by the Adolescent Crisis Team included assessment, short-term crisis intervention and stabilization, intensive family-oriented treatment, case management, group treatment, referral, and case coordination. The Respite House served as a residential home for up to two youth and acted as a diagnostic center, holding environment, and treatment milieu.

The South Shore Mental Health Center implemented no formal evaluation process based on outcome measures; however, agency data revealed an 89% reduction in adolescent admissions to the state hospital psychiatric unit during the 2-year period after the development of the Adolescent Crisis Team. Statistics for 1984–1988 revealed that hospital admissions remained relatively stable, whereas admissions to the Respite House increased.

Transitional Residence Independence Service (TRIS)

An extensive overview of the Children's Crisis Intervention Service (CCIS) was presented by Goldman (1988). CCIS, a community-based residential program, provided crisis intervention and stabilization services to youth in southern New Jersey. This crisis service was a component within the system of care for youth developed by the Transitional Residence Independence Service (TRIS), a psychiatric rehabilitation agency serving children, youth, and adults in the state. Services provided by CCIS included psychiatric evaluation; individual, group, and family counseling; education, recreation, and skill building activities; case management and advocacy services; and referral services. As is true for a majority of crisis programs, no formal evaluation component existed. However, descriptive statistics were provided on the number of youth who were stabilized in the least restrictive setting and returned to community-based placements after discharge. In 1987, 61% of youth who received services returned to their homes. A total of 12% of the youth were placed in foster homes in which the majority received intensive specialized counseling through TRIS, whereas 20% were placed in other residential settings, such as group homes or residential treatment centers. The remaining 7% were hospitalized. A 10% recidivism rate for youth returning for at least one other placement was reported.

In 1988, the Children's Mobile Outreach (CMO) program, a program designed to provide immediate crisis intervention in the client's home or community, was created as an additional service component within TRIS. A team of mental health professionals arrived at the site of the crisis, and psychiatric and psychosocial interventions were employed. Once stabilization was reached, a short-term plan of action was designed. Additional in-home counseling sometimes followed the initial crisis response, and clients were linked to other community service providers. Moore (1991) presented preliminary data from a retrospective analysis of 243 client charts for the period of July 1, 1988, to December 31, 1989. Findings revealed that, for an 18-month period, 76% of the clients who received maximum outreach services from the Children's Mobile Outreach were diverted from placement in a hospital setting. For those who received assessment and minimal crisis intervention, almost 39% of the clients referred were diverted from hospitalization. Of the total sample, 68% were diverted from further entrance into the mental health acute care system.

Since this initial investigation, dramatic changes have taken place in the mental health system of southern New Jersey. As a result of these changes, the CMO program has begun to serve a different population and to provide services to clients discharged from acute care or hospital settings. To examine the effectiveness of the CMO program with these changes in effect, a retrospective survey was conducted from the records of all clients served and discharged during a 12-month period (January 1992–December 1992) (Moore, 1993). Client stability and residential status at discharge were examined for the clients ($N = 192$). Furthermore, a 6-month follow-up telephone survey was completed for a portion of the sample (59 of 83 attempted contacts; 71%). With regard to stability at time of discharge, 68% of *all* clients served were considered stable. The percentage of clients viewed as stable was higher for those receiving crisis services than for those receiving only assessment services. Placement at time of discharge also was examined. Overall, almost 81% of the clients were diverted from hospitalization, whereas only 19% had an inpatient admission. Again, those receiving only assessment services were admitted at much greater rates than those receiving crisis services. At 6-month follow-up, a large percentage remained stable and maintained their community residence. Only 3% of those contacted at follow-up were hospitalized, and only 7% were admitted to a CCIS residential unit.

Huckleberry House

Huckleberry House, a private, nonprofit organization, was founded in 1970 to provide emergency shelter, crisis counseling, and long-term counseling to children and families (Goldman, 1988). The primary mission of Huckleberry House focused on assisting runaway youth to regain control over their lives, to facilitate the building of communication and understanding between youth and adults, and to prevent subsequent runaways and further deterioration of the family relationship. Huckleberry House provided an array of services, including shelter and crisis counseling programs; a voluntary long-term counseling program for adolescents and their families, which included aftercare services; and follow-up services. Information and referral services; educational programs for community groups; and training for volunteers, peer counselors, and students in the human services professional programs also were available.

Information on the clients served as well as documentation of staff and agency activities was gathered. Outcome data on the approximately 700 youth served each year indicated that 53% of these youth returned to the primary family home and 18% were placed in another home setting. A total of 7% were placed in institutional settings, and 6% were placed through the children's service agency. A legal alternative was achieved in 85% of the cases. A total of 7% of the youth were not admitted to the program, and another 7% returned to the streets. In over 75% of the cases, youth engaged in efforts with a parent or parents to improve communication and seek solutions to their problems. Of the 47% referred, over half of the families participated in aftercare services. A total of 46% had no contact with the juvenile justice system, whereas 19% had brief contact only. Information on 77% of the youth was gathered through follow-up telephone calls. This information revealed that 83% had no subsequent episodes of running away from home. About 5% returned to Huckleberry House on multiple occasions.

Systemic Crisis Intervention Program
The Systemic Crisis Intervention Program (SCIP) at the Houston Child Guidance Center, an outpatient treatment program for suicidal children and adolescents, strives to restructure

the client's family and social network. The occurrence of the crisis situation is used as an opportunity to assist the family in learning about the "inherent crisis-intervening potential of their natural networks" (Gutstein et al., 1988, p. 202).

Initial contact with the family in crisis was typically conducted by telephone. After telephone contact, a 3-hour evaluation was conducted and short- and long-term goals were determined. Then families (including extended families) were prepared for crisis gatherings that consisted of two 4-hour meetings in which crisis team members and family members attempted to develop a process of reconciliation among family members to prevent future crisis-provoking situations. After crisis intervention, families were referred for additional outpatient therapy.

Gutstein and Rudd (1990) conducted a study to examine the safety and effectiveness of SCIP. Participants were 47 children and adolescents accepted for treatment by SCIP. Results revealed that, of the children participating in the study, two engaged in suicidal behavior within 6 months of treatment; however, physical harm was minimal. No suicide attempts were made during treatment. There were no reports of injury to either the clients or family members during treatment or the follow-up period. At the outset of treatment, the majority of parents rated their child's presenting problems as "severe" or "catastrophic," but only a small number reported these same ratings after treatment. Adaptive behavior measures also suggested gradual improvement during follow-up. As measured by a problem checklist, the number of problem episodes did not increase following treatment, and, in fact, a significant reduction in problem episodes was revealed over the 18-month follow-up period. Furthermore, ratings of family and marital functioning improved during the 2 years following treatment and were significantly better than pretreatment ratings. With regard to institutional use, only one child had contact following treatment. This number represented significantly fewer children having institutional contacts than for the year prior to treatment.

Outreach

Outreach, a community-based program for adolescents, ran a crisis line and dealt with 231 crisis situations over a 2-year period (Sawicki, 1988). Initial client contact was made by telephone, when an overview of the situation was provided and a meeting site was determined, either the site of the crisis or a neutral site. During the initial meeting, Outreach workers assisted the client in determining precipitating events and developing a short-term plan of action. Intervention usually lasted for about 3 weeks, and further therapy was recommended on an as-needed basis.

Data revealed that, of the 231 calls received by Outreach, almost 200 of those clients were deemed in need of additional therapy. Of those, 174 (87%) made appointments and kept them. Follow-up data indicated that 164 (82%) of those clients who began therapy continued to receive some form of therapy after 30 days. Of the total 231 calls, only 18 (8%) repeated during the 2-year period. Based on these findings, the author concluded that the majority of youth and families treated by the Outreach program showed signs of decreased conflict in a short period of time and displayed a greater willingness to receive assistance from more traditional types of services.

Continuous-Care Model of Crisis Intervention

Stelzer and Elliott (1990) described a continuous-care model of crisis intervention for children and adolescents in operation at the Health Sciences Center in Winnipeg, Manitoba. The model allowed the patient in crisis to be hospitalized briefly and provided continuous care for up to 1 year after admission. After a child was admitted, an intake meeting was arranged between the child, family, school, assessment intervention team, and other relevant agencies. Following the intake meeting, an interdisciplinary assessment was conducted and the crisis was redefined based on these data. Recommendations were presented at a discharge meeting. Follow-up meetings with the family were conducted to examine the child's degree of adaptation to the discharge situation and to resolve any family problems that may have surfaced during the assessment process.

Outcome data revealed that only 8.7% of the yearly population served through the continuous-care model were readmitted. Furthermore, measures of satisfaction indicated that parents and children reported a high degree of satisfaction with most aspects of the program.

Therapeutic In-Home Emergency Services (TIES)

TIES, located in Canton, Ohio, was designed to prevent the out-of-home placement of children with serious emotional and behavioral disturbances. The program consisted of an intensive 6-week in-home intervention that provided crisis intervention and family therapy services. Pastore, Thomas, and Newman (1991) presented the results of a 3-year study designed to examine the effectiveness of the program in effecting changes in individual and family functioning and to compare these effects with programs cited in the literature. The study involved 50 at-risk children and adolescents and their families who received the intensive 6-week home-based intervention. Measures of individual and family functioning were obtained at admission, discharge, and 3 months post-discharge.

Results revealed that 45 of the youngsters remained at home for the duration of the 1-year follow-up period. This placement prevention rate (90%) was found to be significantly higher than rates cited in the literature. Furthermore, an analysis of the measures of individual and family functioning found an improved level of overall functioning. These improvements were maintained at the 3-month follow-up.

Mobile Crisis Team

The Mobile Crisis Team (Child Guidance Center of Greater Cleveland), a 24-hour program, was designed to reduce the unnecessary psychiatric hospitalization of children and youth through the provision of mental health crisis intervention and short-term case management services. The program also used a voucher system that allowed the family to access a range of other services. The mobile crisis unit had two overall purposes: to serve children and youth with serious emotional disorders who were in crisis or at risk of hospitalization and to reduce the need for institutional placement by expanding the range of available placement options. The Mobile Crisis Team strived to treat and stabilize children and youth in their community or natural environment whenever possible. Interventions ranged from telephone consultation to on-site consultation. Case management services were provided to link youth and their families to needed resources in the community.

Gazley (1991) reported the results of a comparison of the percentage of children in crisis referred for hospitalization prior to the establishment of the program and after the implementation of the program. The baseline percentage was 29%. In the first year of operation, the rate of children referred for hospitalization dropped to 6%; in the second year, it dropped to 5%. While these findings are encouraging, conclusive statements regarding the effectiveness of the program await more rigorous research.

Youth Emergency Services (Mobile Crisis Team)

Shulman and Athey (1993) provided a description of Youth Emergency Services (YES), a collaborative mental health service in New York designed to respond to the psychiatric emergencies of children and families through a multisystem, collaborative approach. The overall goal of YES was to provide intensive services to families in an effort to reduce out-of-home placement. Through YES, children and families could begin with any one of the participating agencies and access the resources of the other agencies and the community. YES was comprised of six basic components:

1. Child Crisis Specialists, who screened and evaluated all incoming referrals and linked the family to the appropriate YES component or other agency
2. The Mobile Crisis Team, comprising clinicians who were routed directly to the scene of the crisis, where they attempted to stabilize the situation and conduct an on-site assessment
3. Expanded Children's Services, which consisted of a telephone consultation service regarding areas such as diagnosis, treatment, and medication
4. Home Based Crisis Intervention Services
5. Short-term, out-of-home placement
6. Psychiatric hospitalization

Data indicated that approximately 250 emergency room visits and out-of-home placements were prevented as a result of the Mobile Crisis Team component. A more extensive evaluation of the clinical and cost effectiveness of the program is being conducted.

Home Crisis Intervention Program

Bishop and McNally (1993) presented outcome data for an intensive short-term, home-based crisis intervention program for children and families in Buffalo, New York. The program was designed to stabilize the immediate crisis, prevent hospitalization, and teach families new ways to resolve and prevent future crises. The program provided crisis intervention, case management, and collateral services, such as telephone and interpersonal contacts to link the client to another agency.

A total of 46 children and families were referred to the program during 1989. Of this number, a total of 30 families completed the program as planned. Of the 15 families responding to the inquiry made at 3 months postdischarge, none of the children were reported as having experienced a psychiatric hospitalization during this period. Follow-up reports of eight families at 1 year indicated that no psychiatric or out-of-home placements had occurred.

Scattered-Site Crisis Beds (Suffolk County, New York)

In an effort to provide short-term residential alternatives to hospitalization without the addition of new funding, the Long Island county of Suffolk implemented an interagency model for providing emergency short-term residential services for children and youth in serious crisis through the use of a pool of beds already being administered by the agencies participating in the interagency children's coalition. Due to the nature of the crisis bed program, all referrals are handled by an interagency crisis consultation team. The team was responsible for screening referrals, conducting a brief intake, and presenting this information to the team representative. The representative determined the appropriateness of the referral, selected the most appropriate type of crisis bed for the child, selected the lead agency and case manager, and ensured the establishment and implementation of a disposition plan at the end of the placement period.

An evaluation of the program's effectiveness has been conducted for the period of June 1991 to April 1993 and included a sample of 100 children and youth (Schweitzer & Dubey, 1994). The evaluation yielded four relevant findings. First, youth were successfully placed in community-based residential settings that were not mental health settings but functioned as such with proper supports. Of those placed in the crisis beds, 85% were referred from psychiatric emergency rooms, mobile crisis teams, and treatment and case manager services specifically designed for youth with serious emotional disorders. About 60% of these had a history of inpatient psychiatric hospitalization and exhibited such symptoms as aggression, suicidal ideation, running away, and substance abuse.

Second, the crisis bed program was able to operate efficiently enough to return the youth home or to a longer-term placement within 14 days of referral, the maximum expected length of stay for the program. For the sample ($N = 100$), the median length of stay was 13 days. Greater than 80% were discharged in 15 days or less. Third, the program was able to divert youth from inpatient services. Only 6 of the 100 youth required an inpatient hospitalization during the crisis placement, and 3 were hospitalized within 1 month after discharge from the crisis program. In addition, inpatient admissions to the state children's psychiatric center for the county in which the program was based were reduced by 20% after the establishment of the program. Finally, the cost of the program compared favorably to long-term placements. The crisis bed program was found to operate at about 10% of the cost of hospitalization.

Home Based Crisis Intervention

Of the 697 youth who have completed the Home Based Crisis Intervention (HBCI) program since its inception in 1989, 4.9% required hospitalization during the program (Boothroyd, Evans, & Armstrong, 1995). Based on the Homebuilders model developed in Tacoma, Washington, there are currently eight HBCI programs operating across the state of New York. The goal of this community-based emergency care program is to prevent the hospitalization of youth by providing short-term, intensive, in-home emergency services to families with youth experiencing a psychiatric crisis. After an average length of stay in HBCI of 36 days, 95% of the youth are re-ferred to or enrolled in other services. Nearly 75% of the youth are receiving one service; 15%, two services; and 5%, more than two services.

On the basis of reports from program staff, the eight pro-grams can be classified into three broad categories in terms of their operational orientation: those programs embodying a therapeutic orientation, those programs incorporating a case management orientation, and those programs adhering more strictly to the Homebuilders orientation (i.e., cognitive/behavioral). In an analysis of program orientation and length of stay, results indicated that youth in programs that used a case management approach had shorter lengths of stay by about 2 weeks. A second analysis was performed on length of stay and program staffs' classification of the programs' availability to community resources. The results indicated that those programs considered to have greater access to community resources began discharging sooner and there-fore, on the average, had shorter lengths of stay.

CONCLUSIONS AND FUTURE RESEARCH NEEDS

Crisis services range from residential to nonresidential set-tings and vary with respect to services, personnel, and agen-cies involved. Despite this variability, the underlying goals of most crisis programs are to begin treatment immediately, to provide brief and intensive treatment, to assist in problem solving and goal setting, to involve families in the treatment process, and to assist in the development of a network of community resources for the child and family (Stroul & Friedman, 1986).

As most crisis programs have no formal evaluation com-ponent, few controlled studies examining the effectiveness of crisis and emergency services have been conducted. It has been suggested that this lack of research is due to limited resources to conduct research, a lack of research-oriented cri-sis staff, and the nature of the crisis services that focus on assisting those in extreme distress (Stroul & Goldman, 1990).

Of the evaluations included in the present review, most examined out-of-home placement prevention rates or the percentage of reduction in admissions to residential settings as outcome criteria. The TIES program (Pastore et al., 1991) reported a 90% placement prevention rate, and the continuous-care model of crisis intervention in operation in Winnipeg, Manitoba, related a readmission rate of only 8.7% (Stelzer & Elliott, 1990). The Children's Crisis Intervention Service (Goldman, 1988) reported that 61% of the children returned to their homes, and the Children's Mobile Outreach program (Moore, 1991) reported that 76% of the children had been diverted from hospitalization. A subsequent investigation of the Children's Mobile Outreach program (Moore, 1993) revealed that 81% were diverted from hospitalization, and at 6-month follow-up only 3% of those contacted were hospitalized and only 7% were admitted to a CCIS residential unit. In their examination of a scattered-site crisis bed program, Schweitzer and Dubey (1994) reported that only 6 of the 100 youth in their sample required an inpatient hospitalization during their crisis placement and 3 were hospitalized within 1 month after discharge from the crisis program. This rate of hospitalization during the crisis program is similar to the results of Boothroyd et al. (1995), who report a 4.9% hospitalization rate for youth admitted to the Home Based Crisis Intervention programs operating throughout the state of New York.

In addition to out-of-home placement prevention rates, a few investigations have included measures of individual and family functioning and behavioral indicators as outcome criteria. The most extensive evaluation of additional outcomes was conducted by the Systemic Crisis Intervention Program (Gutstein et al., 1988). Results indicated that children experienced fewer suicidal attempts and aggressive outbursts during treatment and follow-up. Presenting problems were found to decrease, and an improvement in adaptive behavior functioning was evident during follow-up. Problem episodes decreased during follow-up, and family and marital functioning improved.

Moore's investigation (1993) of the Children's Mobile Outreach program found that 68% of all clients served by the program were considered stable at time of discharge, and a large percentage remained stable at 6-month follow-up.

Stroul and Goldman (1990) have suggested that additional research evaluating the effectiveness of crisis interventions and treatment across multiple dimensions is needed, as well as comparisons of different treatment approaches. More research is also needed that explores the differences between crisis-oriented, home-based services and other types of community-based crisis services and considers their roles within a system of care. Finally, investigations comparing the costs of the various crisis and emergency services models are needed, as well as investigations of cost-effectiveness.

REFERENCES

Bishop, E., & McNally, G. (1993). An in-home crisis intervention program for children and their families. *Hospital and Community Psychiatry, 44*(2), 182–184.

Boothroyd, R.A., Evans, M.E., & Armstrong, M.I. (1995). Findings from the New York State home based crisis intervention program. In C.J. Liberton, K.K. Kutash, & R.M. Friedman (Eds.), *The 7th Annual Research Conference Proceedings, A System of Care for Children's Mental Health: Expanding the Research Base* (pp. 25–30). Tampa: University of South Florida, Florida Mental Health Institute, Research and Training Center for Children's Mental Health.

Gazley, C. (1991). Program description: The Mobile Crisis Team Child Guidance Center of Greater Cleveland. In A. Algarin & R.M. Friedman (Eds.), *The 3rd Annual Research Conference Proceedings, A System of Care for Children's Mental Health: Building a Research Base* (pp. 315–325). Tampa: University of South Florida, Florida Mental Health Institute, Research and Training Center for Children's Mental Health.

Goldman, S.K. (1988). *Series on community-based services for children and adolescents who are severely emotionally disturbed. Volume II: Crisis services.* Washington, DC: Georgetown University Child Development Center, National Technical Assistance Center for Children's Mental Health.

Gutstein, S.E., & Rudd, M.D. (1990). An outpatient treatment alternative for suicidal youth. *Journal of Adolescence, 13*(3), 265–277.

Gutstein, S.E., Rudd, M.D., Graham, J.C., & Rayha, L.L. (1988). Systemic crisis intervention as a response to adolescent crises: An outcome study. *Family Process, 27*(2), 201–211.

Moore, J.M. (1991). Children's Mobile Outreach: An alternative approach to the treatment of emotionally disturbed children and youth. In A. Algarin & R.M. Friedman (Eds.), *The 3rd Annual Research Conference Proceedings, A System of Care for Children's Mental Health: Building a Research Base* (pp. 301–313). Tampa: University of South Florida, Florida Mental Health Institute, Research and Training Center for Children's Mental Health.

Moore, J.M. (1993, October). *Emergency psychiatric intervention: Children's Mobile Outreach.* Paper presented at the 3rd Annual Virginia Beach Con-

ference: Children and Adolescents with Emotional or Behavioral Disorders, Virginia Beach, VA.
Pastore, C.A., Thomas, J.V., & Newman, I. (1991). Therapeutic in-home emergency services. In A. Algarin & R.M. Friedman (Eds.), *The 3rd Annual Research Conference Proceedings, A System of Care for Children's Mental Health: Building a Research Base* (pp. 293–299). Tampa: University of South Florida, Florida Mental Health Institute, Research and Training Center for Children's Mental Health.
Sawicki, S. (1988). Effective crisis intervention. *Adolescence, 23*(89), 83–88.
Schweitzer, R., & Dubey, D.R. (1994). Scattered-site crisis beds: An alternative to hospitalization for children and adolescents. *Hospital and Community Psychiatry, 45*(4), 351–354.
Shulman, D.A., & Athey, M. (1993). Youth emergency services: Total community effort, a multisystem approach. *Child Welfare, 72*(2), 171–179.
Stelzer, J., & Elliott, C.A. (1990). A continuous-care model of crisis intervention for children and adolescents. *Hospital and Community Psychiatry, 41*(5), 562–564.
Stroul, B.A., & Friedman, R.M. (1986). *A system of care for children and youth with severe emotional disturbances* (rev. ed.). Washington, DC: Georgetown University Child Development Center, National Technical Assistance Center for Children's Mental Health.
Stroul, B.A., & Goldman, S.K. (1990). Study of community-based services for children and adolescents who are severely emotionally disturbed. *Journal of Mental Health Administration, 17*(1), 61–77.

Residential Services

Psychiatric Hospitals and Residential Treatment Centers

According to Stroul and Friedman (1986), a range of both residential and nonresidential services is necessary within the children's mental health service system. A variety of services along the continuum of care have been established to meet the mental health needs of children and youth. At the most restrictive end of this continuum are residential services, including residential treatment centers (RTCs) and inpatient hospitals.

Inpatient hospitalization is the most restrictive setting along the continuum of care (Tuma, 1989). During hospitalization, the child is removed from the home and the total care of the child is undertaken by hospital staff. This service is "reserved for extreme situations, for youngsters who are showing serious acute disturbances or particularly perplexing and difficult ongoing problems" (Stroul & Friedman, 1986, p. 59). Hospitals use an array of interventions, including individual, family, and group therapy; pharmacotherapy; milieu therapy; and behavioral modification. In addition to those interventions listed above, Dalton, Muller, and Forman (1988) indicate that treatment planning, parent training, and daily school experiences also exist within the hospital setting.

RTCs serve as an alternative to psychiatric hospitalization. These 24-hour facilities, which are not licensed as hospitals, offer mental health services to children (Tuma, 1989). RTCs vary in degree of structure, with some being highly structured, whereas others are similar to group homes or halfway houses. They also vary with regard to the range of services provided. Some offer a full range of services, and others provide only custodial care. Stroul and Friedman (1986) provide a more descriptive definition of RTCs.

Due to the movement toward the establishment of a continuum of care and the increasing concern about the number of children being placed in residential treatment (Wells, 1991), the placement of children in highly restrictive settings has been a focus of attention since the late 1980s. This concern has focused primarily upon ensuring that only those youth who require a highly restrictive placement are placed in residential settings and that an array of alternative services are available to those children who can be adequately served in a less restrictive setting. Because some children do require a highly restrictive placement setting, residential treatment services remain an integral component of a comprehensive system of care for children with serious emotional disorders (Allen & Leichtman, 1990; Singh, Landrum, Donatelli, Hampton, & Ellis, 1994).

ESTIMATES OF SERVICE USE

Due to the various methods used to place youth in residential settings, the number of children receiving such treatment for any given year is uncertain (Yelton, 1993) but appears to be increasing. For example, the Select Committee on Children, Youth, and Families (1990) reported that 25,334 children were in residential care in 1986, which indicated an increase of more than 30% over a 3-year period.

Zimmerman (1990), summarizing survey findings reported by the National Institute of Mental Health, stated that rapid increases in the admission of adolescents to psychiatric hospitals have occurred across the United States. During 1980, over 81,000 youth under the age of 18 were admitted for inpatient psychiatric treatment, and about 55,000 of these individuals fell into the age range of 15–17 years.

The Invisible Children Project was conducted as an effort to gather information on a national level regarding the number of children in residential placement settings as well as the cost of such placements. Based on data from 50 states, Zeigler-Dendy (1990) and Garrison (1990) reported the following summary findings of residential service use from this project: A total of 22,472 children and youth were placed in state hospitals, with an average length of stay of about four months; a total of 4,098 children and youth were placed in out-of-state treatment facilities; and over 14,000 were served in residential treatment facilities within states.

In a paper reviewing mental health service use by adolescents in the 1970s and 1980s, Burns (1991) reported 1986 cross-sectional data for 10- to 18-year-olds. The majority (69%) received outpatient services; the more restrictive settings, such as inpatient, residential treatment centers, and partial hospitalization facilities, served a smaller percentage. In addition, Burns conducted an investigation of service use over time (1975–1986) and found that both outpatient services and residential treatment centers had over a 60% increase in use.

A 1995 report by the American Psychiatric Association (Weller, Cook, Hendren, & Woolston, 1995) concurs that there was a sharp rise in private inpatient treatment from the mid-1980s to the mid-1990s, but suggests that data trends indicate a possible drop in inpatient care rates and lengths of stay during the late 1980s and early 1990s. In an analysis of five states that showed marked decreases in the number of youth hospitalized in state inpatient mental hospitals, the authors concluded that the decrease in child inpatient admissions was not the result of a decrease in population, "but probably resulted from state policy changes connected with the movement of the states toward coordinated 'child centered, family focused' planned systems of care funded by grant programs under the State Comprehensive Mental Health Services Plan Act and the CMHS/NIMH Child and Adolescent Service System Program (CASSP)" (Weller et al., 1995, p. 14).

ESTIMATES OF SERVICE COST

In addition to representing the most restrictive form of care for children, residential services also are the most expensive. Burns and Friedman (1990) stated that psychiatric hospitalization often costs around $500 per day. With an average length of stay of approximately 30 days, this form of treatment can be expensive. Residential treatment centers also are an expensive form of treatment, with costs ranging between $100 and $300 per day of care (Stroul & Friedman, 1986).

Costs estimated from the Invisible Children Project (Garrison, 1990; Zeigler-Dendy 1990) revealed an average per diem rate of about $112 for residential treatment programs. A total annual cost of over $200,000,000 was estimated for the 4,098 children reported in out-of-state residential placement, using cost data from the state of Indiana in the calculation. Based on detailed cost data from six states, the average daily rate for youth in state mental hospitals was about $300; thus, annual treatment costs per child would be $109,193. Based on these cost estimations, it was projected that, on a national basis, treatment for the 22,472 youth in state hospitals with an average length of stay of 4.2 months would cost over $850,000,000. In a 1994 survey of the financial practices of all 50 states, 42 reported the use of state hospitals as a placement for children and youth (Kutash, Rivera, Hall, & Friedman, 1994), indicating that more costly placements are being utilized by most states to some extent.

Discussions on the financing of mental health services for children and youth have suggested that the establishment of a comprehensive continuum-of-care system would result in a dramatic reduction in the cost per child when costs are averaged for all children receiving services along the continuum (Behar, 1990). This point is further emphasized by the findings of a study conducted by Hoagwood and Cunningham (1992) in which cost estimates suggested that the implementation of a comprehensive array of services could reduce state residential and inpatient psychiatric hospitalization costs by 60%. Promising results from the California AB377 Evaluation Project have begun to demonstrate that the implementation of a comprehensive system of care can result in overall cost savings (Attkisson, Dresser, & Rosenblatt, 1995; Rosenblatt, Attkisson, & Fernandez, 1992). This project, which replicated the system of care for youth with serious emotional disorders pioneered in Ventura County, has been implemented in three other California counties. Due to the high numbers of youth served in residential group homes and the subsequent cost of serving these youth, the project sought to reduce placements and costs by providing a coordinated and effective system of care. Results indicated that the demonstration counties, when compared with the state of California as a whole, reduced the number of group home placements and thus expenditures.

Similar results were obtained for the CHAMPUS Tidewater Demonstration Project (Burns, Thompson, & Goldman, 1992). This project was an attempt to reduce the use of more restrictive and costly residential services through the implementation of a partial hospitalization placement setting and a more effective monitoring system. Results revealed a shift in the use of levels of care, with a greater number of children being admitted to the outpatient treatment setting over time, whereas admissions to inpatient treatment settings decreased over time. Thus, as the use of more costly inpatient treatment settings declined, the costs of mental health services decreased.

EFFECTIVENESS AND OUTCOME RESEARCH

Along with issues of cost and appropriate use of residential care for children, there has been attention to the effectiveness of this type of care. The need for efficacy research was emphasized by Dalton et al. (1988):

> Recent pressure from third party payors, as well as philosophical and theoretical changes within the field of mental health, have raised questions about the appropriateness of psychiatric hospitalization of children. Increased scrutiny has underscored the need for efficacy studies to determine the utility of this form of treatment. (p. 232)

However, little research on outcomes and effectiveness of residential treatment is available (Burns & Friedman, 1990; Stroul & Friedman, 1986). The studies that do exist can be categorized into four broad types, based on the research strategy or design used. First, the majority of studies conducted have used single samples that analyzed changes in functioning from the beginning of treatment to the end of treatment (pre–post designs). Some studies examined the efficacy of different treatment strategies used within residential settings, and others compared residential treatment with no-treatment groups. The final type consisted of studies that compared residential services with alternative types of services. Studies falling into each of these four categories are described within this chapter.

Although residential treatment centers and inpatient hospitalization differ, the majority of studies and reviews in the research literature examine both residential treatment and hospitalization. Furthermore, both forms of care focus on providing long-term (as opposed to acute or crisis care), intensive, 24-hour care. Therefore, for the purpose of this chapter, research on residential treatment centers and inpatient hospitalization is reviewed together.

Descriptive Studies

Blotcky, Dimperio, and Gossett (1984) summarized the findings of 24 efficacy studies conducted between 1936 and 1982 that examined the outcome of children treated in psychiatric hospitals. The following factors were found to be predictive of a positive outcome: adequate intelligence, nonpsychotic diagnoses, no clear signs of neurological dysfunction, absence of bizarre and antisocial behaviors, healthy family functioning, adequate length of stay, and adequate aftercare. Most of the studies suffered from serious methodological weaknesses; thus, findings should be viewed with caution.

Pfeiffer and Strzelecki (1990) provided a review of outcome studies on inpatient psychiatric and residential treatment of children and youth conducted from 1975 to 1990. It should be noted that none of the 34 follow-up studies in this review utilized random assignment of subjects (Bickman, 1992). A synthesis of the results of the 34 follow-up and outcome studies was conducted using a method developed by the authors. For a discussion of possible limitations of this technique, see Blotcky and Dimperio (1991). For each study, the relationship between outcome and a predictor variable was rated as negative, neutral, or positive; this value was then adjusted according to the sample size. Using this method, the following factors were found to be predictive of a positive outcome: the presence of a specialized treatment regimen, the availability of aftercare services, and less severe child and family dysfunction. Intelligence and length of stay were moderately predictive of a favorable outcome. Age and gender were found to be unrelated to outcome.

Two additional single-sample outcome studies have been described in the literature. One of four studies reviewed by

Burns and Friedman (1990) revealed the effectiveness of a residential treatment center and found postdischarge support to be necessary for the maintenance of treatment gains. One of two studies described by Dalton et al. (1988) was an outcome study that measured the effectiveness of specific inpatient interventions in the treatment of children with conduct disorder and antisocial behavior ($N = 26$). The results indicated no significant change in behavior following 3 months of treatment on a psychiatric unit, although some gains in social relationships were noted.

Yet another review of the available outcome research on the residential treatment of children and youth has been rendered by Curry (1991). In his review of studies using single-sample designs, Curry included both hospital-based and residential treatment-based studies. The results of the hospital-based studies suggested that outcomes vary. Whereas many children improve, others show no improvement, and a small percentage may reveal "seriously negative outcomes" (p. 350) at follow-up. The importance of support and aftercare following discharge was emphasized. Curry then summarized the findings of three residential treatment-based studies. Briefly, the first study found that subjects' adaptation improved during treatment and that the majority (71%) were functioning adequately at follow-up. The second study revealed an association between adaptation after discharge and the child's perception of support and continuity. A third study demonstrated that, whereas most of the children treated in the residential treatment center showed improvement during treatment, treatment gains were not predictive of later adjustment.

A number of descriptive studies conducted from 1988 to 1995 and not included in previous reviews are described here in greater detail. Ney, Adam, Hanton, and Brindad (1988) conducted a 1-year follow-up study to determine the effectiveness of a child psychiatric unit. After inpatient treatment, changes in the functioning of parents and children involved in the study ($N = 112$) were assessed. The majority of parents indicated that they were more frequently able to talk and to listen to their child. At 1 year postdischarge, about 84% of the parents reported that the program was very helpful, 8%

reported that treatment made no difference, and 4% indicated that problems had escalated as a result of the program. Of the families, 64% indicated that the whole family was managing better as a result of treatment. The parents indicated that they became angry, lost control, or criticized their children on a less frequent basis and reported the acquisition of more effective discipline skills. Although some were not statistically significant, outcome measures for the children revealed changes in the positive direction. A large improvement in the number of police contacts was not found; however, the number of children involved in this behavior was minimal. Significant changes in the five scales of the Peterson-Quay Behavior Problems Checklist were noted. Of the children, 97% returned to the families from which they were admitted. A 2% readmission rate was observed over the 3-year history of the program.

A 1-year follow-up report on the effects of long-term hospital treatment of children and adolescents was conducted by Berland and Safier (1988). Subjects were patients at the Children's Hospital of The Menninger Clinic, a long-term treatment facility. Patients ($N = 42$) were grouped into three major diagnostic categories: psychoses, personality disorders, and neuroses. Results obtained from telephone interviews with youth and parents revealed that more than two thirds had a positive outcome at 1 year follow-up, and almost 75% of those with personality disorders had improved.

Blumberg (1992) conducted a study to assess the general treatment effects of an inpatient/day program unit of a children's psychiatric hospital. Subjects ($N = 115$) exhibited serious emotional and/or behavioral problems that required a restrictive environment. Results of a standardized behavior checklist completed by parents and teachers at admission and at 3 months, 6 months, and 12 months postdischarge revealed that the children's behavior tended to improve following treatment in the hospital. Poor initial response to treatment as well as a diagnosis of attention-deficit/hyperactivity disorder (ADHD) was predictive of poor outcome.

A more recent follow-up study was conducted to determine short-term outcomes for children ($N = 65$) discharged from a child psychiatric unit (Kalko, 1992). Outcomes were

Table 6.1. Overview of studies examining the effectiveness of residential services

Author or reviewer	Type of article	Design	Results/conclusions
Blotcky, Dimperio, & Gossett (1984)	Summarized 24 outcome studies conducted between 1936 and 1982	Outcomes of psychiatric hospitalization; single-sample design	Factors predictive of positive outcome: adequate IQ, nonpsychotic diagnoses, no neurological impairments, absence of bizarre and antisocial behaviors, healthy family functioning, adequate length of stay, and adequate aftercare
Pfeiffer & Strzelecki (1990)	Reviewed and assessed outcome of 34 studies conducted between 1975 and 1990 that examined inpatient psychiatric and residential treatment of children	34 follow-up single-sample studies	Factors found to be predictive of positive outcome: standardized treatment regimen; aftercare services; less severe child and family dysfunction Factors found to be moderately predictive of positive outcome: higher IQ levels and longer stays in a residential facility
Burns & Friedman (1990)	Reviewed results of 4 studies	One an RTC follow-up study, single-group design	Generally positive results; postdischarge support necessary to maintain treatment gains
Dalton, Muller, & Forman (1988)	Reviewed two outcome studies of inpatient treatment	Single sample design: outcome of children receiving treatment for conduct disorder and antisocial behavior	After 3 months of inpatient treatment, some gains in social relations as measured on a behavioral rating scale, but no significant change in other behaviors

(continued)

115

Table 6.1. *(continued)*

Author or reviewer	Type of article	Design	Results/conclusions
Curry (1991)	1) Reviewed hospital-based studies 2) Summarized 3 residential treatment-based studies	1) Single-sample designs 2) Single-sample design and follow-up	1) Outcomes varied; many improved, others experienced no improvement, and a small percentage displayed negative outcomes. Support and aftercare services are important. 2a) Improved during treatment and majority were functioning adequately at follow-up. 2b) An association was found between adaptation after discharge and the child's perception of support and continuity. 2c) Most children showed improvement during treatment; treatment gains were not predictive of long-term adjustment.
Ney, Adam, Hanton, & Brindad (1988)	Examined effectiveness of a child psychiatric unit (N = 112)	One-year follow-up study	Majority of parents were more frequently able to talk and listen to child. At 1-year follow-up, 85% viewed the program as helpful, 8% reported that treatment made no difference, and 4% reported that problems increased following treatment. 64% indicated greater family functioning. Outcome measures for the children revealed changes in the positive direction. 97% of the children returned to their families. A 2% readmission rate was observed over the 3-year history of the program.

Berland & Safier (1988)	Examined long-term hospital treatment of children and youth ($N = 42$) at Children's Hospital of The Menninger Clinic	1-year follow-up study	More than 2/3 of the group had a positive outcome at 1-year follow-up, and almost 75% of those with personality disorders improved.
Blumberg (1992)	Examined effectiveness of an inpatient/day program unit of a children's psychiatric hospital ($N = 115$)	Single-sample study	Children's behavior tended to improve after treatment in the hospital. Poor initial response as well as a diagnosis of ADHD were predictive of poor outcome.
Kalko (1992)	Investigated short-term outcomes for children ($N = 65$) discharged from a child psychiatric unit	Single-sample, follow-up study	No significant effects by follow-up or length of stay. Poor short-term outcome was predicted by a diagnosis of ADHD, older age at admission, child depression or sadness, neurological or psychotic symptoms, limited aftercare services, history of physical abuse, and higher intellectual functioning. Parents reported a more positive adjustment at home. Services did not differ as a function of the child's perceived improvement.
Parmelee et al. (1995)	Examined factors for 90 youth during hospitalization and at 3 months and 12 months postdischarge	Single sample, follow-up study	There was a decline in placement stability for youth at the 12-month postdischarge follow-up. The most influential predictors of successful outcome at discharge were living with a family member at the time of hospitalization and the participation of the family in treatment during hospitalization.

(continued)

Table 6.1. (continued)

Author or reviewer	Type of article	Design	Results/conclusions
Hoagwood & Cunningham (1992)	Presented outcome data for students (N = 114) placed in residential treatment for educational purposes	Single-sample, outcome study	In 25% of the cases, a positive outcome was revealed (returned to school or school-related vocational training). Over 60% experienced no or minimal progress or were discharged with a negative outcome (running away). In 11% of the cases, students remained in residential placement but made progress. Positive outcomes were associated with shorter lengths of stay (less than 15 months).
Cornsweet (1990)	Reviewed 2 controlled studies of inpatient treatment	Problem-solving skills training vs. relationship treatment vs. attention control group	At discharge and follow-up, improved behavioral gains for problem-solving skills training group as compared with groups receiving relationship therapy and control group.
Curry (1991) and Quay (1986)	Reviewed 4 studies	1) Between-program study using between-treatment groups 2) Within-program study using a between-treatment design	1) No major difference found between groups receiving transactional analysis and behavior modification treatment approaches. 2) Those in the authority-based treatment group committed fewer offenses than those in the self-governing group.
Dalton, Muller, & Forman (1988)	Reviewed 2 outcome studies of inpatient treatment	Skills training vs. no-treatment control	Skills-based treatment group receiving treatment in inpatient setting exhibited less aggression and externalizing behaviors than did no-treatment control group.

Study			
Curry (1991) and Quay (1986)	Reviewed 4 studies	Between-program study using treatment–no-treatment groups	Those receiving treatment fared better than the no-treatment group; only 50% received a change in their special education placement category of severely behaviorally impaired.
Burns & Friedman (1990)	Reviewed 4 studies	1) Randomly assigned to treatment and control groups 2) RTC vs. alternative treatment method 3) RTC vs. alternative treatment method	1) No difference between groups at discharge. At follow-up, hospitalized youth were twice as likely to be in institutions. 2) No significant benefits from residential treatment when compared with alternative treatment. 3) No significant benefits from residential treatment when compared with alternative treatment.
Cornsweet (1990)	Reviewed 2 controlled studies of inpatient treatment	Hospital vs. hospital-based evaluation/intensive community-based treatment	Both groups improved on behavioral and educational variables; family functioning remained constant.
Curry (1991) and Quay (1986)	Reviewed 4 studies	Across-program study design	For those youth deemed as in need of residential care, results revealed a lower rate of re-arrest for those receiving residential treatment than for those receiving community-based treatment.

RTC, residential treatment center.

However, since the mid-1980s the service delivery field has experienced a shift in this perception of intensity; that is, appropriate levels of intensive service can be rendered in the child's natural environments through the providing of family preservation and individualized, wraparound services. Thus, home- and community-based approaches as well as residential services are now considered to be appropriate avenues for the provision of intensive services (Knitzer, 1993).

Studies on the outcomes and efficacy of residential treatment of children vary widely in their focus and methodology. The majority of research studies presented in the current review did not examine residential care in comparison with other service approaches, but rather were descriptive in nature. Due to the nature of single-sample designs, these studies failed to address the question of effectiveness but did contribute to the existing knowledge base. Factors found to be predictive of positive outcome included adequate intelligence, nonpsychotic diagnoses, no clear signs of neurological impairment, the absence of bizarre and antisocial behaviors, healthy family functioning, adequate length of stay, and adequate aftercare (see Blotcky et al., 1984). Based on their review of 34 studies, Pfeiffer and Strzelecki (1990) found the following factors to be related to a positive outcome: a standardized treatment regimen, aftercare services, and less severe child and family dysfunction. Length of stay and IQ were found to be moderately predictive of positive outcome. Parmelee et al. (1995) found that residing with a family member at admission and having parental involvement during treatment were factors predictive of a positive outcome. Hoagwood and Cunningham (1992) found that shorter lengths of stay were associated with positive outcomes.

Other studies have documented factors found to be predictive of poor outcome. Blumberg (1992) found that a diagnosis of attention-deficit/hyperactivity disorder (ADHD) and poor initial response to treatment were associated with poor outcome. Kalko (1992) also found that a diagnosis of ADHD was predictive of poor outcome, as well as older age at admission, child depression or sadness, neurological or psychotic symptoms, limited aftercare services, history of physical abuse, and higher intellectual functioning.

Other studies included in this review compared residential treatment services to no-treatment groups. Generally, these studies (Curry, 1991; Dalton et al., 1988) found that youth receiving residential services experienced more positive outcomes than did youth receiving no services.

A limited number of studies examined the effectiveness of residential services as compared with other methods of service delivery (Burns & Friedman, 1990; Cornsweet, 1990; Curry, 1991). Currently, no conclusive evidence exists to support the effectiveness of residential treatment over other service types.

Despite the wide variability among residential treatment programs and a lack of rigorously controlled studies, residential treatment services have been found to result in improved functioning for *some* children. Residential treatment plays a significant role in the treatment of children and youth with serious emotional disturbances. However, considerable research is needed before conclusive statements regarding the effectiveness of residential services can be drawn. Future research efforts must concentrate on determining which youth can most benefit from this type of treatment and which treatment approaches work best with specific populations.

Despite the significantly higher cost of residential placement in comparison with other service types and the criticisms that have characterized it as an overused and unnecessarily restrictive placement setting, this component continues to be an integral part of a comprehensive system of care as it continues to serve as a necessary placement for a portion of children and youth identified as having an emotional or a behavioral disorder (Singh et al., 1994).

REFERENCES

Allen, L.G., & Leichtman, M. (1990). Introduction. *Bulletin of the Menninger Clinic, 54*(1), 1–2.

Attkisson, C.C., Dresser, K., & Rosenblatt, A. (1995). Service systems for youth with severe emotional disorder: System of care research in California. In L. Bickman & D. Rog (Eds.), *Children's mental health services: Research, policy, and innovation* (pp. 236–280). Beverly Hills: Sage Publications.

Behar, L. (1990). Financing mental health services for children and adolescents. *Bulletin of the Menninger Clinic, 54*(1), 127–139.

Berland, D.I., & Safier, E.J. (1988). One-year follow-up report on long-term hospital treatment of children and adolescents. *Bulletin of the Menninger Clinic, 52*(2), 145–149.

Bickman, L. (1992). Designing outcome evaluations for children's mental health: Improving internal validity. In L. Bickman & D. Rogs (Eds.), *Evaluating mental health services for children* (pp. 57–68). San Francisco: Jossey-Bass.

Blotcky, M.J., & Dimperio, T. (1991). Outcome of inpatient treatment (Letters to the editor). *Journal of the American Academy of Child and Adolescent Psychiatry, 30*(3), 507.

Blotcky, M.J., Dimperio, T.L., & Gossett, J.T. (1984). Follow-up of children treated in psychiatric hospitals: A review of studies. *American Journal of Psychiatry, 141*, 1499–1507.

Blumberg, S. (1992). Initial behavior problems as predictors of outcome in a children's psychiatric hospital. In A. Algarin & R.M. Friedman (Eds.), *The 4th Annual Research Conference Proceedings, A System of Care for Children's Mental Health: Expanding the Research Base* (pp. 185–188). Tampa: University of South Florida, Florida Mental Health Institute, Research and Training Center for Children's Mental Health.

Burns, B.J. (1991). Mental health service use by adolescents in the 1970s and 1980s. *Journal of the American Academy of Child and Adolescent Psychiatry, 30*(1), 144–150.

Burns, B.J., & Friedman, R.M. (1990) Examining the research base for child mental health services and policy. *Journal of Mental Health Administration, 17*(1), 87–98.

Burns, B.J., Thompson, J.W., & Goldman, H.H. (1992). Initial treatment decisions by level of care for children in the CHAMPUS Tidewater Demonstration. In A. Algarin & R.M. Friedman (Eds.), *The 4th Annual Research Conference Proceedings, A System of Care for Children's Mental Health: Expanding the Research Base* (pp. 209–222). Tampa: University of South Florida, Florida Mental Health Institute, Research and Training Center for Children's Mental Health.

Cornsweet, C. (1990). A review of research on hospital treatment of children and adolescents. *Bulletin of the Menninger Clinic, 54*(1), 64–77.

Curry, J.F. (1991). Outcome research on residential treatment: Implications and suggested directions. *American Journal of Orthopsychiatry, 61*(3), 348–357.

Dalton, R., Muller, B., & Forman, M. (1988). The psychiatric hospitalization of children: An overview. *Child Psychiatry and Human Development, 19*(4), 231–244.

Garrison, P. (1990). Invisible Children report summary. In A. Algarin, R.M. Friedman, A.J. Duchnowski, K. Kutash, S.E. Silver, & M.K. Johnson (Eds.), *Second Annual Conference Proceedings on Children's Mental Health Services and Policy: Building a Research Base* (pp. 359–371). Tampa: University of South Florida, Florida Mental Health Institute, Research and Training Center for Children's Mental Health.

Hoagwood, K., & Cunningham, M. (1992). Outcomes of children with emotional disturbance in residential treatment for educational purposes. *Journal of Child and Family Studies, 1*(2), 129–140.

Kalko, D.J. (1992). Short-term follow-up of child psychiatric hospitalization: Clinical description, predictors, and correlates. *Journal of the American Academy of Child and Adolescent Psychiatry, 31*(4), 719–727.

Knitzer, J. (1993). Children's mental health policy: Challenging the future. *Journal of Emotional and Behavioral Disorders, 1*(1), 8–16.

Kutash, K., Rivera, V.R., Hall, K.S., & Friedman, R.M. (1994). Public sector financing of community-based services for children with serious emotional disabilities and their families: Results of a national survey. *Journal of Mental Health Administration, 21*(3), 262–270.

Ney, R.G., Adam, R.R., Hanton, B.R., & Brindad, E.S. (1988). The effectiveness of a child psychiatric unit: A follow-up study. *Canadian Journal of Psychiatry, 33,* 793–799.

Parmelee, D.X., Cohen, R., Nemil, M., Best, A.M., Cassell, S., & Dyson, F. (1995). Children and adolescents discharged from public psychiatric hospitals: Evaluation of outcome in a continuum of care. *Journal of Child and Family Studies, 4*(1), 43–55.

Pfeiffer, S.I., & Strzelecki, S. (1990). Inpatient psychiatric treatment of children and adolescents: A review of outcome studies. *Journal of the American Academy of Child and Adolescent Psychiatry, 29*(6), 847–853.

Quay, H.C. (1986). Residential treatment. In H.C. Quay & J.S. Werry (Eds.), *Psychopathological disorders of childhood* (3rd ed., pp. 558–582). New York: John Wiley & Sons.

Rosenblatt, A., Attkisson, C.C., & Fernandez, A.J. (1992). Integrating systems of care in California for youth with severe emotional disturbance. II: Initial group home expenditure and utilization findings from the California AB377 Evaluation Project. *Journal of Child and Family Studies, 1*(3), 263–286.

Select Committee on Children, Youth, & Families, U.S. House of Representatives. (1990). *No place to call home: Discarded children in America.* (HR #101-395). Washington, DC: Author.

Singh, N.N., Landrum, T.J., Donatelli, L.S., Hampton, C., & Ellis, C.R. (1994). Characteristics of children and adolescents with serious emotional disturbance in systems of care. Part I: Partial hospitalization and inpatient psychiatric services. *Journal of Emotional and Behavioral Disorders, 2*(1), 13–20.

Stroul, B.A., & Friedman, R.M. (1986). *A system of care for children and youth with severe emotional disturbances* (rev. ed.). Washington, DC: Georgetown University Child Development Center, National Technical Assistance Center for Children's Mental Health.

Tuma, J.M. (1989). Mental health services for children: The state of the art. *American Psychologist, 44*(2), 188–199.

Weller, E.B., Cook, S.C., Hendren, R.L., Woolston, J.L. (1995). *On the use of mental health services by minors: Report to the American Psychiatric Association Task Force to study the use of psychiatric hospitalization of minors: A review of statistical data on the use of mental health services by minors.* Washington, DC: American Psychiatric Association, Office of Minority Affairs.

Wells, K. (1991). Placement of emotionally disturbed children in residential treatment: A review of placement criteria. *American Journal of Orthopsychiatry, 61*(3), 339–347.

Yelton, S. (1993). Children in residential treatment—Policies for the '90s. *Children and Youth Services Review, 15*(3), 173–193.

Zeigler-Dendy, C.A. (1990). The Invisible Children Project: Methods and findings. In A. Algarin, R. Friedman, A. Duchnowski, K. Kutash, S. Silver, & M. Johnson (Eds.), *Second Annual Conference Proceedings on Chil-*

dren's Mental Health Services and Policy: Building a Research Base (pp. 353–358). Tampa: University of South Florida, Florida Mental Health Institute, Research and Training Center for Children's Mental Health.

Zimmerman, D.P. (1990). Notes on the history of adolescent inpatient and residential treatment. *Adolescence*, 25(97), 9–38.

CHAPTER 7

Family Support Services

The field of children's mental health is experiencing a "quiet revolution" in the design, delivery, and evaluation of services for children with emotional, behavioral, or mental disorders and their families (Friesen, 1993). This period of transition has been described as "a shift in both conceptualization and practice" (Duchnowski & Kutash, 1993, p. 2). This evolving mental health service delivery system for children and families is characterized by a number of factors, one of which is the full participation of families in every phase of the treatment planning process (Knitzer, 1993). Instead of the historical practice of blaming families for the problems experienced by their children, advocates, researchers, and policy makers now agree on the necessity of parent and family involvement in the provision of mental health services to children and adolescents. Whereas some have argued that parental involvement should occur because of its positive effect on outcomes for children and families, others have proposed that the process itself has "intrinsic value and that it satisfies an ethical obligation to parents and families in our society" (Heflinger, 1995, p. 6). Regardless of the rationale for family involvement, family participation is a crucial component in the delivery of mental health services to children and adolescents.

Along with this emerging role of the family as partners in their child's mental health treatment is the acknowledgment of the need to develop family support services. Family support programs provide a wide array of services designed to assist families in meeting their emotional, social, and basic needs. Families of children with emotional and behavioral disorders are faced with a number of complex issues that go well beyond the everyday challenges of family life, including disruptions in communication patterns, family roles, and patterns of daily living; the unpredictability of the child's cognitive and emotional development; a sense of loss as the expectations of the parents fail to be commensurate with the abilities of the child; concerns of long-term care and support, which alter the roles of the parents and siblings; and the need for additional coping strategies and resources for the management of stress (Modrcin & Robinson, 1991). These issues clearly illustrate the need to develop efforts to provide families with much-needed support and resources.

Because of the recency of the family support movement for families of children with emotional and behavioral disorders and hence the lack of literature in this area, this chapter draws from the available literature on family support services for other populations as well. In addition, literature on family support/self-help groups is included because of its inherent relationship with the area of family support. Thus, the primary purpose of this chapter is to review the literature on the effectiveness of family support services and to summarize the literature on outcomes associated with participation in family support/self-help groups for families with children who have emotional and behavioral disorders. To serve as a comparative group of studies, the literature on the effectiveness of both family support programs and family support/self-help groups is reviewed for families whose members have an illness or disability. Finally, a description is given for a select segment of the effectiveness literature on family support services for *all* families, regardless of situation, including programs that have a communitywide focus and those geared toward at-risk families, as well as those with a focus on families in general. Although a complete review of family support services with a communitywide focus is beyond the scope of this chapter, a few examples of this type of effort are provided to demonstrate the wide diversity among family support services and program efforts.

OVERVIEW OF FAMILY SUPPORT SERVICES

Family Support Programs

Family support programs vary along a number of dimensions, including the range and intensity of services offered;

populations targeted; and operational, organizational, and structural factors. However, the common thread among them appears to be their primary focus on providing services to families that "empower and strengthen adults in their roles as parents, nurturers, and providers" (Weissbourd & Kagan, 1989, p. 21).

In the realm of family support services for families of children with emotional and behavioral disorders, "family support is doing whatever it takes to make it possible for families that include members with disabilities to just be families" (Agosta, 1992, p. 4). The primary goal of family support services is "to keep families together and to help all family members to achieve balanced lives" (Friesen & Wahlers, 1993, p. 12). Until the mid-1980s, the concept of family support services was restricted to the provision of respite services (i.e., providing a period of relaxation to the parents or child). Currently, services within the domain of family support may include

> family self-help, support and advocacy groups and organizations; information and referral; education that will support families in becoming active, informed decision-makers on behalf of their family and the child; advocacy with and on behalf of the family, if needed; the capacity to individualize, provide flexible support services, and meet unplanned needs quickly and responsively; in-home and out-of-home respite care, with an emphasis on neighborhood and community participation for the child and conceptualized not as a clinical service but as a support for the whole family; cash assistance; assistance with family survival needs (housing, food, transportation, home maintenance, etc.); and other supports, as determined by the family. (Federation of Families for Children's Mental Health, 1992, p. 1)

Family Support/Self-Help Groups

Family support and self-help groups represent *only one* of the possible components that constitute family support services. In the system of care model proposed by Stroul and Friedman (1986), self-help and support groups fall under the rubric of operational services, defined as a range of support services that "cross the boundaries between different types of services" and play a critical role in the "overall effective operation of the system" (p. 93). The primary focus of these groups is to provide emotional support and practical assistance to members who share a common problem or concern (e.g., disability, substance abuse, bereavement).

Support groups for families of children with emotional or behavioral disorders appear to be expanding. Although there is wide variation in the membership, format, and duration of these groups, most share common characteristics (Koroloff & Friesen, 1991). Usually, 4–20 parents meet on a regular basis to discuss the problems and issues associated with parenting a child with emotional and behavioral disorders and to provide mutual encouragement and suggestions for dealing with problematic situations. Groups may serve as an information resource, an opportunity to promote the importance of legal and legislative action on behalf of children, and a chance for families who are experiencing similar situations or conditions to share common concerns and provide mutual support. Furthermore, groups may be informal or formal in nature; that is, "they may be formally constituted and affiliated with larger formal organizations or may involve relatively informal meetings of a small number of family members" (Koroloff & Friesen, 1991, p. 267).

EFFECTIVENESS AND OUTCOME RESEARCH

Services for Families of Children with Emotional and Behavioral Disorders

Family Support Programs Since 1984, when the first local-level, parent-run groups began forming, significant progress has been made in the organization of parent support efforts (Friesen & Koroloff, 1990). The first local, parent-run organization for families of children and adolescents with emotional disturbances was the Parents Involved Network (PIN), sponsored by the Mental Health Association of Southeastern Pennsylvania. This organization provides a number of parent support services, including support groups, telephone information, newsletters, referral services, and advocacy training (Karasik & Samels, 1990). PIN served as a model for other parent-run organizations, and as a result a number of similar programs have emerged across the country.

Although a number of programs exist, research on the effectiveness of family support services for families of children with emotional and behavioral disorders is scarce (Frie-sen & Koroloff, 1990; Zigler & Freedman, 1987). Despite this paucity of research, some evaluative studies have been con-ducted to assess the benefits of family support services for families of children with emotional disorders and other spe-cial needs. In a brief review of these studies, Friesen and Ko-roloff (1990) stated that a considerable research base existed for family support services designed for prevention and early intervention with children and families at risk, as well as for services provided to families of children with a variety of disabilities. The positive effects of these family support ser-vices have been shown primarily in the areas of specific ser-vices, such as respite care and the use of social support systems. The benefits of respite care included positive bene-fits for siblings, a reduction in the family's sense of isolation, and decreases in the incidence of child abuse and neglect. Parent support groups have been found to result in an in-crease in access to information and improved problem-solving abilities for a portion of parents. Furthermore, family members have been found to hold more positive attitudes, take a more optimistic outlook on parenting, and hold a more positive view of their children's behaviors (see Friesen & Ko-roloff, 1990).

Agosta (1992) reported the results of evaluations of fam-ily support services in two states. The determination of ef-fectiveness was based on placement preference and on meeting family needs. The placement preferences of the fam-ilies participating in four pilot programs in Illinois were ex-amined. Results revealed little overall change in placement preference over time; however, few families preferred an out-of-home placement for their child *before* receiving family sup-port services. To assess the effectiveness of family support services in meeting family needs, evaluations of pilot pro-grams in Illinois and a statewide program in Iowa were con-ducted. Evaluation results revealed that families indicated a high degree of satisfaction with the family support programs and reported that the programs had a favorable impact on various family life domains. Although families indicated that many needs were left unmet, results revealed a significant reduction in family needs in areas specifically addressed by the family support program.

The Finger Lakes Family Support Project, a professional family-support program for families of children with emotional problems, operates as a collaboration between professionals and family members in nine rural counties in the Finger Lakes area of New York State (Friesen & Wahlers, 1993). The project consists primarily of three major components: family-support groups; child care and respite care; and conferences, family retreats, and training opportunities. An evaluation of the program revealed that many parents felt that the project assisted them in decreasing stress, increasing their ability to cope and to help themselves, and keeping their children at home. Furthermore, stress associated with parenting and the parents' perception of the severity of their children's problems decreased over time (Murray, 1992).

Support/Self-Help Groups The needs of families of children with serious emotional disorders vary; however, emotional support appears to be a common component. In fact, in a national study of parents whose children had emotional and behavioral disorders, Friesen (1990) found that 72% indicated that emotional support was the activity most helpful in coping with the difficulties associated with raising their child.

Although a small number of support groups for parents of children with emotional and behavioral disorders have been in existence for a number of years, research on the effectiveness and outcomes of these groups is scant. A review of the literature conducted by Koroloff and Friesen (1991) revealed no studies that specifically addressed the effectiveness of support groups for parents of children with emotional disorders. Although a limited amount of research is available, there exists a widespread belief that participation in parent support groups leads to beneficial outcomes for members. Some of these benefits have been identified as the acquiring of 1) information about the disorder and available services, 2) advocacy information, 3) problem-solving skills, 4) emotional support, 5) reduced isolation, and 6) assistance with coping (Gartner, cited in Koroloff & Friesen, 1991). These benefits of participation in support groups have been described in the literature (see Koroloff & Friesen, 1991, for a brief review). The following section presents a description of the available literature on the outcomes associated with participation in self-help/support groups for families of children with emotional and behavioral disorders.

In a study involving 834 parents of children with emotional disorders, a written questionnaire was distributed to compare parents who participated in parent support groups with nonmembers across a number of variables (Koroloff & Friesen, 1991). Results revealed no significant differences between members and nonmembers on most demographic variables; however, members of support groups reported that they needed and used more information and services than nonmembers but found these more difficult to locate than did nonmembers. Most important, 31% of all respondents identified involvement with other parents of children with serious emotional disorders as the most helpful activity in increasing their ability to cope with raising their child.

Sheridan and Moore (1991) reported the results of a six-session educational and support group for parents of adolescents with schizophrenia. The goals of the group were to increase parents' level of knowledge about schizophrenia and to provide group support to decrease the parents' sense of isolation. Two questionnaires, designed to assess the impact of the illness on group members as well as parents' level of knowledge about the disorder, were administered during the initial group session. At termination, a third questionnaire was administered to obtain feedback on the group process. The responses of 29 parents from two groups were used in the analysis. With regard to the impact of the disorder on the family, results indicated that the areas most affected were relaxation time and the ability to concentrate on work at home or in a job. In general, participants, and especially mothers, indicated that they worried too much. Furthermore, results indicated that attitudes about discipline had changed with regard to their child with schizophrenia. Most participants related that their family was open and able to discuss emotions, with feelings of worry and sadness being the most difficult to express and feelings of anger and happiness the least difficult to express.

No significant difference in pretest and posttest scores was evident for parents' level of knowledge about schizophrenia. This may be attributed to the fact that parents scored very high on the pretest measure and thus had little room for improvement. Feedback indicated that support from other parents in similar situations was the aspect most valued by participants. The impression of the clinical team was that participation in the group and confidence in a group setting was "matched" by gains in the parents' ability to manage their children's behavior in the home. The team also reported the receipt of fewer crisis telephone calls from parents during and after participation in the group.

Dreier and Lewis (1991) presented the results of the evaluation of an open-ended group for parents of children hospitalized for mental illness. The group model consisted of a combination of the support and psychoeducational group models. The goals of the group were to assist parents in feeling less apprehensive about the hospitalization of their child and to decrease feelings of failure in their parenting role. Outcome evaluation was based on staff observations of parent–child interaction and anecdotal reports from parents. Parents reported that they experienced more positive feelings about themselves and their ability to understand and interact more competently with their children.

PIN, a self-help, advocacy, information, and training resource, was established "to provide a vehicle through which parents of children with serious emotional problems can raise their concerns and voice their collective priorities" (Corp & Kosinski, 1991, p. 241). In a study conducted to investigate the outcomes of parent involvement in support group and advocacy training activities, Fine and Borden (1992) found that participation in the self-help group met parents' support needs; and participation in training activities allowed them to become more effective advocates for their children. The parents' perceptions of the changes in their lives as a result of their participation in the support group revealed two important outcomes. The first was a change in their reactions to a crisis situation; that is, during a crisis, parents continued to attend group meetings and to interact in an effective manner with other parents by giving and receiving support. A second outcome involved an increase in self-esteem; although initially these parents perceived themselves as failures and poor parents, involvement with PIN resulted in a greater sense of control and self-assurance, thus decreasing feelings of guilt and blame for their child's difficulties. At follow-up, the majority (72%) of parents continued to have some form of interaction with PIN, and 44% of these parents were involved in either support group activities or advocacy efforts on a regular basis. In another review of PIN, Corp and Kosinski (1991) found that parents who were in contact with parent groups on a frequent basis were able to gain more desirable and effective services for their children and reported a marked reduction in feelings of isolation, guilt, and anger.

Moynihan, Forward, and Stolbach (1994) reported the results of a consumer satisfaction survey of 96 parents of children and adolescents with serious mental disturbance in Colorado. Although not designed to measure client outcome, the consumer satisfaction surveys provided valuable information about the concerns and needs of families. In the area of parent support/self-help groups, 36% of those surveyed indicated that they had participated in a parent support or self-help group. Of these, 70% indicated that the group was an effective vehicle for meeting their needs. The remaining parents indicated that they were unsure or did not believe that participation in a support group met their needs.

Heflinger (1995) summarized the results of the Vanderbilt Family Empowerment Project, which examined the effectiveness of a parent support curriculum designed to promote parent–professional partnerships in children's mental health services. Using an experimental research design, parents ($N = 253$) who agreed to take part in the study were randomly assigned to the parent groups or to a control group. Data were gathered at pretest and at 3 and 12 months posttest using the Vanderbilt Mental Health Services Efficacy Questionnaire. This questionnaire measures a parent's belief that he or she could engage in those activities necessary to affect how his or her child was treated and the belief that, if he or she did engage in these activities, this would lead to more appropriate treatment and, ultimately, more positive outcomes for his or her child. At follow-up, those parents participating in the parent empowerment group revealed a significant increase in knowledge of the mental health system and of mental health services efficacy.

Services for Families of Children with an Illness or Disability

Family Support Programs The Center for the Development of Informal Education (CEDIN) is a family support program that seeks to promote and strengthen families by offering training opportunities in prenatal, early childhood, and parenting education. Services are community-based, family-centered, and culturally comprehensive in nature. The primary aspect of the Center is the home-based Parent-Child Program, which instructs parents in the use of various methods for preventing or reversing developmental delays in their infants and toddlers. A 3-year evaluation (Allen, Brown, & Finlay, 1992) of the CEDIN program revealed positive effects for the children in the areas of health and development. At age 2, the children in the CEDIN program were slightly more advanced in their mental development than those in a comparison group. These children also experienced fewer hospitalizations as they aged, possibly due to the emphasis on health education. Furthermore, program participants improved in the areas of discipline methods and the safety and appearance of their living environment.

Support/Self-Help Groups In 1985, Hinrichsen, Revenson, and Shinn conducted an empirical investigation of peer support groups for individuals with scoliosis and their families. Data on psychosocial outcomes and satisfaction with services were obtained from survey questionnaires in a cross-sectional study of adults with scoliosis and adolescents with scoliosis and their parents, each of whom were members of a self-help organization for persons with scoliosis ($n = 245$). Nonparticipants who had expressed an interest in scoliosis groups ($n = 495$) served as a comparison group. Data revealed that, although most participants reported a high degree of satisfaction with the group, participation had little effect on psychosocial outcomes. Participation seemed to be most helpful for adult patients, particularly those who had endured the most intensive medical treatment.

Moran (1985) evaluated the impact of participation in an early intervention program for mothers (N = 85) of children with disabilities. Findings indicated that, in comparison to nonparticipants, mothers in the program reported less intensive levels of stress; however, no differences in informal support network development were noted.

A study involving mothers (N = 56) of children with special needs was conducted by Shapiro (1989). Interview data revealed that those who participated in support groups (n = 34) were less depressed, perceived their child as less burdensome, and employed more problem-solving coping strategies than did mothers who did not participate in support groups (n = 22).

Krauss, Upshur, Shonkoff, and Hauser-Cram (1993) examined the impact of participation in parent groups on mothers of infants with disabilities (N = 150). Results revealed that intensity of participation was associated with both positive and negative outcomes in the areas of maternal functioning and social support. Participation in the parent group was associated with significant increases in the size and helpfulness of social support networks; however, increased group attendance was also related to increased levels of personal strain and greater adverse effects on familial and social relationships.

In an evaluation of a bimonthly group program for fathers of children with disabilities, Vadasy, Fewell, Meyer, and Greenberg (1985) found lower levels of stress and depression and a higher degree of satisfaction for both parents following the fathers' group participation for a period of 1 year. Follow-up results revealed that the effects were maintained over time; however, fathers reported a higher degree of pessimism over time (Vadasy, Fewell, Greenberg, Dermond, & Meyer, 1986).

James and Egel (1986) investigated the impact of direct prompting and modeling procedures on the interactions between children without disabilities (n = 3) and their preschool-age siblings with disabilities involved in a play group. Results revealed that the intervention was effective in increasing positive reciprocal interactions between the siblings and that these positive interactions generalized to larger play groups across settings. Follow-up data at 6 months revealed that positive behaviors were maintained over time.

McLinden, Miller, and Deprey (1991) examined the effects of a 6-week support group for siblings ($n = 6$) of children with special needs. Pretest and posttest assessments revealed that the support group had a significant positive effect on perceptions of social support for participants as compared with those in the control group ($n = 5$). No significant differences were noted on outcome measures assessing behavior problems, self-concept, or knowledge and attitudes. Parental interview data revealed some improvements in participants' behavior toward siblings.

Services with Communitywide
Focus for At-Risk and Other Families

Reis, Bennett, Orme, and Herz (1989) conducted a quasi-experimental evaluation of three demonstration family support programs implemented in 1982. The primary goal of each family support program was to increase parent competency and to reduce the rate of child abuse and neglect on a communitywide basis. Respondents included a total of 365 mothers who participated in the family support programs and 265 matched controls. Treatment outcomes included measures of level of depression, perceived social support, knowledge of child development, and punitive parenting attitudes. Although the programs offered a diverse array of services, each had a drop-in center for parents and offered parent education and support classes. Two of the sites also offered a home visitors program. Results revealed little relationship between the receipt of family support services and treatment outcome measures.

In 1985, an evaluation of four pilot Parents as Teachers (PAT) programs in Missouri revealed promising results. The programs were initiated in 1981 and were implemented on a statewide basis in 1984. Operating through the public school system, the programs strived to

> give children the best possible start in life and prepare them for school success by supporting parents in their role as children's first and most important teachers. (Allen et al., 1992, p. 48)

Services are provided to families until the child reaches the age of 3; however, some continue to be involved in other available activities until their child reaches kindergarten. The programs comprise four main components, including home visits, group meetings for parents, regular monitoring of children's health and developmental status, and referral to social service and other agencies when necessary. The 1985 evaluation revealed that the 3-year-old children who had been involved in the program since birth were significantly more advanced than the comparison group in language development, in problem-solving skills and other intellectual abilities, and in the display of coping skills and positive child-adult relationships. Furthermore, children evaluated at the end of their first-grade year were doing better in school than children in the comparison group, and their parents displayed greater involvement in the education of their children. Additionally, teachers reported that children in the PAT program were better prepared for school than most other children in similar families. A 1991 evaluation of the statewide program revealed that the benefits of PAT had been sustained over time. In general, parents experienced improved coping skills, an increase in their knowledge of child development, and an enhanced ability to communicate in an effective manner with their children. Furthermore, the children performed significantly above national norms on achievement, and greater than half of the children with developmental delays had overcome them by age 3.

The Parent Services Project (PSP) evolved as a result of the expansion of child care centers to offer services and support to the entire family. The primary goals of PSP were to increase parents' sense of self-worth, to decrease feelings of isolation, to improve parenting skills, and to assist parents in locating support resources in the community. Available activities included parenting classes, peer support groups, mental health workshops, opportunities for socialization, special groups and activities for fathers, respite child care on weekends, and emergency home-based child care services. During 1985–1988, an evaluation (see Allen et al., 1992) of PSP revealed that, as compared with those in a control group, parents participating in the project experienced significantly lower levels of stress, maintained lower stress levels, and had higher self-esteem. Furthermore, these parents experienced an improvement in their attitudes about child rearing and interactions with their children.

The Maternal Infant Health Outreach Worker Project (MIHOW), a network of family support programs, was established in 1982 to serve rural families in the Mississippi Delta and Appalachian region. The goals of the MIHOW project were to improve prenatal and infant care and to enhance the development of human resources in the region. Outreach services constituted the primary activity of these family support programs. Outreach workers visited families' homes to assist with health and child-rearing problems and to link families with other resources in the community. Early evaluations of the efficacy of the MIHOW programs indicated that maternal health care practices during pregnancy and infant feeding practices were improved and that mothers were more responsive to their children, provided more appropriate play materials, and were more involved in promoting the achievement of age-appropriate skills in their children than before participation in the program. More recent evaluations have incorporated the use of focus groups and in-depth interviews with parents and staff. These evaluations have demonstrated the positive effects of the programs in that parents reported having more hope for the future, more control over their own lives, and an increased ability to advocate for their children (see Allen et al., 1992).

Friends of the Family is an independent agency that oversees a statewide network of family support centers in Maryland. The centers were established to address the problem of high rates of teen pregnancy and an increasing incidence of child abuse and neglect. Programs varied from area to area to meet the needs of the local community; however, *all* programs provided a range of social support services and assistance in child development. General Equivalency Diploma (GED) preparation courses and parenting classes also were offered. In 1988, a total of eight Friends of the Family support centers existed in the state. An evaluation of these programs revealed that the centers were reaching their goal of serving high-risk families. The researchers concluded that "the programs were contributing to a reduced likelihood of repeat pregnancies, clear educational advances by participating mothers, and enhanced family stability" (Allen et al., 1992, p. 66).

The Ewa Healthy Start Program at Ewa Beach in Hawaii began in 1985 and was used as a model for the state-funded Healthy Start/Family Support Services program established in 1988. The purpose of the program was to develop a strategy to prevent juvenile delinquency and other problems associated with an abusive, disadvantaged childhood. Families of newborns are screened for family risk factors, and those with a substantial number of risk factors participate in the program. Families receive weekly visits from a family support worker who links the family with a pediatrician and assists the family in coping with crisis situations (e.g., aids the family in obtaining housing assistance). Home visits also provide support for improved parent–child relationships, increased knowledge of child development, and enhanced parenting skills. Child development specialists are available to assist families of children with special needs. A 3-year evaluation of the Ewa demonstration project revealed positive effects of the program (see Allen et al., 1992). The program appeared to be successful in identifying families at high risk for child abuse or neglect and was successful in the prevention of abuse and neglect. For a total of 241 at-risk families, child abuse was averted in 100% of the cases, and neglect occurred in four cases. For families identified as high risk but not served by the program because of a lack of resources, the rate of abuse was three times higher than in the general population. Outcomes were positive for nine of the Healthy Start/Family Support Services programs in Hawaii, as abuse and neglect each were averted in over 99% of the cases.

Telleen, Herzog, and Kilbane (1989) examined the impact of a family support program on social support, depression, parenting stress, and perceptions of children for mothers ($N = 38$) with children under the age of 7 years. One group ($n = 16$) participated for 3 months in a support group for mothers, and another group ($n = 22$) took part in a parent education class for 3 months. A matched control group ($N = 23$) comprised mothers who used a medical clinic for the pediatric care of their children. After the 3-month period, mothers in both treatment groups reported feeling less social isolation and parenting stress than those in the control group.

McBride (1991) examined the impact of parent education and support programs on paternal involvement and perceptions of parental competence for a sample of fathers. Participants included fathers and their preschool-age children ($N =$ 60) who volunteered to take part in the program. A "wait-list" control group technique was used to assign subjects to two treatment groups and two control groups. Those in the treatment group participated in one of two parent education/ play group programs, each having the major components of group discussions and father–child play time. Pretest and posttest data were gathered from all participants. Results revealed that participation in the program had a significant positive effect on the fathers' perceptions of parental competence and parental involvement in the areas of interaction and accessibility, particularly on non-workdays.

CONCLUSIONS AND FUTURE RESEARCH NEEDS

As families enter into partnerships with professionals in the treatment of their children with special needs, there is an increasing recognition of the need for supportive services for families. A number of family support services and programs have been developed to meet the needs of these families. Family support programs can cater to families of children with a wide variety of special needs and provide a broad array of services, which may include self-help, support, and advocacy groups; information and referral sources; educational and training opportunities; respite care; and cash supplements or assistance with the acquisition of basic needs.

Evaluation findings for the two studies associated with family support services for families with children with emotional and behavioral disorders generally revealed positive outcomes for parents (see Agosta, 1992; Friesen & Wahlers, 1993). The evaluations in this developing area of service delivery revealed that parents who received family support services were satisfied overall with services received; experienced a positive impact on various family life domains;

reported a significant reduction in stress and in family needs in areas specifically addressed by the program; and indicated an increase in coping skills and the ability to maintain their child in the home.

Evaluations of outcomes associated with participation in self-help support groups for families with children who have emotional and behavioral disorders also have shown generally positive results. The results of three studies indicated that a large percentage of parents who participated in a self-help/support group reported emotional support as the most beneficial outcome of their participation (see Friesen, 1990; Koroloff & Friesen, 1991; Sheridan & Moore, 1991). These survey results correspond to the program evaluation results of the PIN program. The results of the two studies of PIN (Fine & Borden, 1992; Corp & Kosinski, 1991) revealed that parent participation in the self-help group met parents' support needs; increased self-esteem; and reduced feelings of isolation, guilt, and anger. Furthermore, the results of this program evaluation found that parents who were frequently in contact with support groups or participated in training activities were able to become more effective advocates and gain desirable services for their children. The remaining studies in this section focused on group models that provided both support and education for parents with children with emotional or behavioral disorders. Findings revealed that parents reported a more positive self-perception and an increased ability to understand and interact with their children in a competent manner (Dreier & Lewis, 1991). Only one of these studies (Heflinger, 1995) was conducted using an experimental design. Results revealed that participants in the experimental group increased not only their knowledge of mental health service delivery but also their self-efficacy in dealing with the mental health service delivery system as compared with a control group.

The investigations of family support programs and support/self-help groups for families of children with an illness or disability again point to the high level of satisfaction with participation. In the one study reviewed on a family support program providing training and education aimed at preventing or reversing developmental delays in infants, participants' children experienced fewer hospitalizations and were slightly more advanced in mental development than a comparison group of children (see Allen et al., 1992). In the area of support/self-help groups, studies that employed the use of a comparison group found positive effects of participation (e.g., decreased levels of stress and depression) but mixed results on psychosocial outcomes and the increase of social support networks (see Hinrichsen et al., 1985; Moran, 1985; Shapiro, 1989). Furthermore, Krauss et al. (1993) found that, although participation was associated with significant increases in the size and helpfulness of social support networks, increased group attendance was also related to elevated levels of personal strain and greater adverse effects on familial/social relationships. An examination of a group for fathers of children with disabilities (Vadasy et al., 1985) found lower levels of stress and depression and a higher degree of satisfaction for both parents after participation in the group. These mixed results possibly point to the varied and individualized needs of parents participating in support/self-help groups. Two studies (James & Egel, 1986; McLinden et al., 1991) focused on the unique support needs of siblings of children with disabilities. Again, these studies point to the varied and unique needs of siblings of children with disabilities.

The review of selected outcomes on family support services with a communitywide focus or a focus on at-risk populations or families in general revealed mixed results. Some of the studies found positive individual outcomes such as school preparedness and increased achievement levels, but outcomes on overarching community indicators varied across studies. These varied outcomes support the caution put forth by Weissbourd (1991) that

> the family resource movement carries with it the destructive potential of *over*-promise and its corresponding danger of diminishing the impact of programs. Programs should not be saddled with the unrealistic expectation that they will solve the macro-level ills that contribute to family crises such as poverty, inadequate housing, and unemployment. What they *can* do is enhance the competency of parents and enable participants to build skills, utilize resources, and develop the confidence necessary to advocate on their own behalf. (p. 70)

As the movement toward family-centered care continues, parents are taking on a variety of alternative roles. According to Friesen and Koroloff (1990), one of the most significant factors in augmenting the role of parents is the formation of an organized and distinct "parent voice" (p. 19). Advocacy is one of the most important roles for parents. In fact, an increase in the advocacy movement has been proposed as one of the major challenges of the 1990s (Duchnowski & Friedman, 1990). Historically, the parents of children with serious emotional disorders have not been "an organized advocacy force" (Friesen & Huff, 1990, p. 32); however, since the late 1980s a number of positive developments in this area have occurred (see Duchnowski & Friedman, 1990; Friedman, Duchnowski, & Henderson, 1989), including the establishment of the Federation of Families for Children's Mental Health, a national parent-run organization that strives to improve services for children with serious emotional disorders and their families.

Another significant development in the area of family involvement has been the occurrence of the "Families as Allies" conferences. Beginning in 1986, these conferences were held in every region of the country to allow parents and professionals to form partnerships and to identify parents of children with serious emotional disturbances who were interested in forming support groups. As a result of these conferences and similar efforts, a number of statewide parent advocacy organizations and local support groups were developed to help parents "organize for the purposes of support, education, and advocacy" (Friesen & Koroloff, 1990, p. 19). Furthermore, a number of national organizations have begun to focus on the needs of children (e.g., the National Mental Health Association, National Alliance for the Mentally Ill, Children's Defense Fund, the Child Welfare League of America, the Association of Child Advocates).

A more recent development has been the availability of statewide family network demonstration grants funded by the Center for Mental Health Services. Grants are to be used for the establishment or enhancement of statewide, family-controlled networks to provide support and information to families of children with serious emotional, behavioral, or mental disorders.

Koroloff, Elliott, Koren, and Friesen (1994) provided a description of yet another alternative role for parents. Based on the principles of parent-to-parent support, the Family Connections Project has implemented Family Associates in three counties in Oregon. The Family Associate is

> a parent without professional mental health training who acts as a system guide to low-income families whose children have been referred to mental health services through Early and Periodic Screening, Diagnosis, and Treatment Program. (p. 240)

The Family Associate provides emotional support, services and referral information, and assistance with transportation and child care. The role of the Family Associate is to assist families in overcoming barriers that may inhibit access to mental health services. An evaluation of the effectiveness of the use of the Family Associate currently is being conducted. The Regional Intervention Program in Tennessee represents yet another approach in which parents of children with behavioral disorders and/or developmental delays have assumed an alternative role in treatment by serving as primary therapists for their children and as trainers and resources to other parents (see Timm, 1993).

The research contained in this review points to a number of possible directions. First, the importance of conducting further research to better document the needs of families is evident. Second, research must focus on how to involve families more fully in the treatment planning process for their children and on how to support them more adequately in their role as "allies" in this process. Third, additional research must ascertain more completely the effects of participation in self-help and support groups for families, parents, and siblings. Fourth, additional information is needed about *which* group approaches and models (e.g., psychoeducational, support) work most effectively with *which* families. Finally, as families continue to take on an increasingly significant role in the treatment of their children with emotional and behavioral problems, it is likewise important that researchers begin to involve families in the research planning process.

REFERENCES

Agosta, J. (1992). Building a comprehensive support system for families. In A. Algarin & R.M. Friedman (Eds.), *The 4th Annual Research Conference Proceedings, A System of Care for Children's Mental Health: Expanding the Research Base* (pp. 3–16). Tampa: University of South Florida, Florida Mental Health Institute, Research and Training Center for Children's Mental Health.

Allen, M., Brown, P., & Finlay, B. (1992). *Helping children by strengthening families: A look at family support programs.* Washington, DC: Children's Defense Fund.

Corp, C., & Kosinski, P. (1991). Parents Involved Network, Delaware County, Pennsylvania Chapter: A self-help, advocacy, information and training resource for parents of children with serious emotional problems. In A. Algarin & R.M. Friedman (Eds.), *The 3rd Annual Research Conference Proceedings, A System of Care for Children's Mental Health: Building a Research Base* (pp. 241–247). Tampa: University of South Florida, Florida Mental Health Institute, Research and Training Center for Children's Mental Health.

Dreier, M.P., & Lewis, M.G. (1991). Support and psychoeducation for parents of hospitalized mentally ill children. *Health and Social Work, 16*(1), 11–18.

Duchnowski, A.J., & Friedman, R.M. (1990). Children's mental health: Challenges for the nineties. *Journal of Mental Health Administration, 17*(1), 3–12.

Duchnowski, A.J., & Kutash, K. (1993, October). *Developing comprehensive systems for troubled youth: Issues in mental health.* Paper presented at the Shakertown Symposium II: Developing Comprehensive Systems for Troubled Youth, Shakertown, KY.

Federation of Families for Children's Mental Health. (1992). *Family support statement.* Alexandria, VA: Author.

Fine, G., & Borden, J.R. (1992). Parents Involved Network Project (PIN): Outcomes of parent involvement in support group and advocacy activities. In A. Algarin & R. Friedman (Eds.), *The 4th Annual Research Conference Proceedings, A System of Care for Children's Mental Health: Expanding the Research Base* (pp. 25–29). Tampa: University of South Florida, Florida Mental Health Institute, Research and Training Center for Children's Mental Health.

Friedman, R.M., Duchnowski, A.J., & Henderson, E.L. (1989). *Advocacy on behalf of children with serious emotional problems.* Springfield, IL: Charles C Thomas.

Friesen, B.J. (1990). National study of parents whose children have serious emotional disorders: Preliminary findings. In A. Algarin, R. Friedman, A. Duchnowski, K. Kutash, S. Silver, & M. Johnson (Eds.), *Second Annual Conference Proceedings on Children's Mental Health Services and Policy: Building a Research Base* (pp. 29–44). Tampa: University of South Florida, Florida Mental Health Institute, Research and Training Center for Children's Mental Health.

Friesen, B.J. (1993). Overview: Advances in child mental health. In H.C. Johnson (Ed.), *Child mental health in the 1990s* (pp. 12–19). (DHHS Publication No. SMA 93-2003). Rockville, MD: U.S. Department of Health and Human Services, Public Health Services, Substance Abuse and Mental Health Services Administration, Center for Mental Health Services.

Friesen, B.J., & Huff, B. (1990). Parents and professionals as advocacy partners. *Preventing School Failure, 34*(3), 31–35.

Friesen, B.J., & Koroloff, N.M. (1990). Family-centered services: Implications for mental health administration and research. *Journal of Mental Health Administration, 17*(1), 13–25.

Friesen, B.J., & Wahlers, D. (1993). Respect and real help: Family support and children's mental health. *Journal of Emotional and Behavioral Problems, 2*(4), 12–15.

Heflinger, C.A. (1995). Studying family empowerment and parental involvement in their child's mental health treatment. *Focal Point, 9*(1), 6–8.

Hinrichsen, G.A., Revenson, T.A., & Shinn, M. (1985). Does self-help help? An empirical investigation of scoliosis peer support groups. *Journal of Social Issues, 41*(1), 65–87.

James, S.D., & Egel, A.L. (1986). A direct prompting strategy for increasing reciprocal interactions between handicapped and nonhandicapped siblings. *Journal of Applied Behavior Analysis, 19*(2), 173–186.

Karasik, J., & Samels, M. (1990). Banding together: Speaking with one voice. *Preventing School Failure, 34*(3), 11–13.

Knitzer, J. (1993). Children's mental health policy: Challenging the future. *Journal of Emotional and Behavioral Disorders, 1*(1), 8–16.

Koroloff, N.M., Elliott, D.J., Koren, P.E., & Friesen, B.J. (1994). Connecting low income families to mental health services: The role of the family associate. *Journal of Emotional and Behavioral Disorders, 2*(4), 240–246.

Koroloff, N.M., & Friesen, B.J. (1991). Support groups for parents of children with emotional disorders: A comparison of members and nonmembers. *Community Mental Health Journal, 27*(4), 265–279.

Krauss, M.W., Upshur, C.C., Shonkoff, J.P., & Hauser-Cram, P. (1993). The impact of parent groups on mothers of infants with disabilities. *Journal of Early Intervention, 17*(1), 8–20.

McBride, B.A. (1991). Parent education and support programs for fathers: Outcome effects on paternal involvement. *Early Child Development and Care, 67,* 73–85.

McLinden, S.E., Miller, L.M., & Deprey, J.M. (1991). Effects of a support group for siblings of children with special needs. *Psychology in the Schools, 28,* 230–237.

Modrcin, M.J., & Robinson, J. (1991). Parents of children with emotional disorders: Issues for consideration and practice. *Community Mental Health Journal, 27*(4), 281–292.

Moran, M.A. (1985). Families in early intervention: Effects of program variables. *Zero to Three, 5,* 11–14.

Moynihan, M.H., Forward, J.R., & Stolbach, B. (1994). Colorado's parents' satisfaction survey: Findings and policy implications for local systems of care. In C.J. Liberton, K. Kutash, & R.M. Friedman (Eds.), *The 6th Annual Research Conference Proceedings, A System of Care for Children's Mental Health: Expanding the Research Base* (pp. 69–79). Tampa: University of South Florida, Florida Mental Health Institute, Research and Training Center for Children's Mental Health.

Murray, J. D. (1992). *Analysis of outcome data of the Finger Lakes family support program.* Mansfield, PA: Rural Services Institute, Mansfield University.

Reis, J., Bennett, S., Orme, J., & Herz, E. (1989). Family support programs: A quasi-experimental evaluation. *Children and Youth Services Review*, *11*(3), 239–263.

Shapiro, J. (1989). Stress, depression, and support group participation in mothers of developmentally delayed children. *Family Relations*, *38*, 169–173.

Sheridan, A., & Moore, L.M. (1991). Running groups for parents with schizophrenic adolescents: Initial experiences and plans for the future. *Journal of Adolescence*, *14*, 1–16.

Stroul, B.A., & Friedman, R.M. (1986). *A system of care for children and youth with severe emotional disturbances* (rev. ed.). Washington, DC: Georgetown University Child Development Center, National Technical Assistance Center for Children's Mental Health.

Telleen, S., Herzog, A., & Kilbane, T.L. (1989). Impact of a family support program on mothers' social support and parenting stress. *American Journal of Orthopsychiatry*, *59*(3), 410–419.

Timm, M.A. (1993). The Regional Intervention Program: Family treatment by family members. *Behavioral Disorders*, *19*(1), 34–43.

Vadasy, P.F., Fewell, R.R., Greenberg, M.T., Dermond, N.L., & Meyer, D.J. (1986). Follow-up evaluation of the effects of involvement in the fathers program. *Topics in Early Childhood Special Education*, *6*, 16–31.

Vadasy, P.F., Fewell, R.R., Meyer, D.J., & Greenberg, M.T. (1985). Supporting fathers of handicapped young children: Preliminary findings of program effects. *Analysis and Intervention in Developmental Disabilities*, *5*, 125–137.

Weissbourd, B. (1991). Family resource and family support programs: Changes and challenges in human services. In D.G. Unger & D.R. Powell (Eds.), *Families as nurturing systems: Support across the lifespan* (pp. 69–85). New York: Haworth Press.

Weissbourd, B., & Kagan, S.L. (1989). Family support programs: Catalysts or change. *American Journal of Orthopsychiatry*, *59*(1), 20–31.

Zigler, E.F., & Freedman, J. (1987). Evaluating family support programs. In S.L. Kagan, D. Powell, B. Weissbourd, & E. Zigler (Eds.), *America's family support programs* (pp. 352–361). New Haven: Yale University Press.

C H A P T E R 8

Case Management/
Service Coordination

The service needs of children with emotional and behavioral disorders and their families are complex and multidimensional, requiring not only the availability of an array of services but mechanisms to ensure that services are provided in a coordinated, cohesive manner. One of the most rapidly developing methods in the effort to coordinate these services is case management, defined as

> a mechanism for linking and coordinating segments of a service delivery system, within a single agency or involving several providers, to ensure the most comprehensive program for meeting an individual client's needs for care. (Austin, 1983, p. 16)

Case management, or service coordination, is designated as an "operational service" within the system of care model because of its importance to the overall effective operation of the system and its tendency to cross the boundaries between different types of services. Case management has been referred to as the "backbone of the system of care" (Stroul & Friedman, 1986) and the cohesive element that holds the system together (Behar, 1985).

Friesen and Poertner (1995) have pointed out that the functions of the case manager/service coordinator can vary depending upon the level (the child, family, or system level) at which the activities occur (see Figure 8.1). They have defined case management as the "activities of a designated person aimed at improving the circumstances of specific children and families," whereas the term service coordination is used to characterize "activities and processes that have implications for a broader set of children and families or for the shape and structure of the service delivery system" (p. xxiv). Within the direct service role, case managers appear to play an especially critical role in implementing individualized ser-

	Purpose of Service Coordination Efforts:			
Level at which activity occurs:	Improving match between client needs and system response	Direct service: Initiation and maintenance of client change	System change	Cost containment
Child and Family (Case)	*Primary*	*Possible*	*Possible*	*Possible*
Systems	*Secondary*	*No*	*Primary*	*Possible*

Figure 8.1. Relationship between the purpose of service coordination efforts and the level at which activities occur. (From Friesen, B.J., & Poertner, J. [1995]. *From case management to service coordination for children with emotional, behavioral, or mental disorders: Building on family strengths* [p. xxii]. Baltimore: Paul H. Brookes Publishing Co.; reprinted by permission.)

vice approaches, including "wrapping" services around each youth and his or her family (Katz-Leavy, Lourie, Stroul, & Zeigler-Dendy, 1992). Furthermore, the role of some case managers has been expanded to include the provision of clinical services. The functions of "clinical case managers" include crisis intervention, medication management, supportive counseling, and individual and family therapy (Stroul, 1995).

The primary role of a case manager is to ensure that needed services are delivered in an effective and efficient manner (Garland, Woodruff, & Buck, 1988). The general functions of a case manager have been outlined as follows:

1. Assessment—an evaluation process to determine needs or problems
2. Service planning—the identification of specific treatment goals and the planning of individualized activities and services needed to achieve goals
3. Service implementation—ensuring that the individualized service plan is executed as intended in a timely, appropriate manner
4. Service coordination—the referral, transfer, or connection of the child to the appropriate services delineated in the treatment plan

5. Monitoring and evaluation—consistent and ongoing contact with the child to ensure that services are being delivered and continue to be appropriate
6. Advocacy—speaking for and representing the needs of the client to secure services and entitlements. (Stroul, 1995)

CASE MANAGEMENT APPROACHES AND MODELS

A number of case management approaches and models have been established. In an effort to provide a case management topology, Robinson (1991) identified four models of case management used for individuals with serious mental illness: the expanded broker model, the personal strengths model, the rehabilitation model, and the full support model. The primary function of the traditional case manager is that of broker with the primary responsibility of making arrangements for clients to receive services within the mental health domain. This is true also of the expanded broker model; however, as the name suggests, the focus expands beyond merely linking clients to mental health services and includes other community resources as well. The personal strengths model of case management addresses the social problems of individuals with serious mental illness. The model emphasizes the identification of the individual's strengths and strives to create situations in which success can be achieved, thus increasing the personal strengths of the individual. Furthermore, individuals are provided with assistance in securing community resources necessary for human growth and development.

The goal of the rehabilitation model is to aid clients in meeting with success and in achieving satisfaction in the social environment of their choice with the least amount of professional assistance required. The rehabilitation model emphasizes the identification and strengthening of the client's skills as well as the identification and evaluation of skill deficits that may serve as barriers to the achievement of personal goals. Individuals are taught the necessary skills to meet their goals. The full support model of case management stresses active involvement as a means of assisting individuals with mental illness to make improvements in their level of functioning in the community and to reduce symptomatology. Case management practices involve teaching clients an array of coping skills and providing support to clients in the community.

Burns, Gwaltney, and Bishop (1995) described seven case management models developed by Weil for either children or adults, each of which could be implemented within a range of minimal to full-scale comprehensive service systems. These models are the generalist/service broker model, the primary therapist model, the interdisciplinary team model, the comprehensive service center model, the family as case manager model, the supportive care model, and the volunteer as case manager model.

Within the generalist/service broker model, the case manager is a human services professional responsible for service coordination for a client. In the primary therapist model, the case manager is usually that professional whose relationship to the client is primarily therapeutic, such as a psychologist, psychiatrist, or master's-level social worker; and case management functions are undertaken as an extension of the therapeutic intervention. The interdisciplinary team model combines the activities of specialists to provide case management functions according to each person's area of expertise. In some cases, one team member assumes primary responsibility for guiding the client through the service system. In the comprehensive service center model, full services are provided; the lead agency provides basic services and linkage to services in other agencies. The family as case manager model uses family members as case managers, whereas the supportive case model uses citizens in rural (and occasionally inner city) areas to deliver mental health services and provide linkage to community supports. Finally, in the volunteer as case manager model, professionally trained volunteers assist clients while under the supervision of those who are legally responsible.

Working from the typologies of case management services for adults set forth by Robinson (1991; see also Robinson & Toff-Bergman, 1989), Early and Poertner (1995) have identified and described the four concomitant practice approaches that have recently been employed with children and families who have emotional and behavioral disorders: outpatient therapy/case management, brokerage, interdisciplinary or interagency team, and strengths-based case management.

Within the outpatient therapy/case management approach, case management functions are added to existing therapeutic personnel within an outpatient therapy program. As the therapist and the child and/or parent see the need for additional services, linkages to other services and agencies are initiated. However, given the limitations of office-based therapy, such linkages are often restricted to passive referrals by the therapist. In the brokerage approach, the main responsibility of the case manager is to make arrangements for clients to receive services. The role of the case manager is to know what services are available to meet the needs of the child and/or family and to coordinate the arrangements necessary for the receipt of services.

Within the two remaining approaches, interdisciplinary team and strengths-based, teams are used to assist and augment the case management function. The interdisciplinary team is often used with children and adolescents with multiple needs who require multiple agencies. The team serves primarily as a coordinating mechanism across the various multiple agencies and services. In some cases, one person is designated as the lead case manager responsible for linking the child and/or family member to services. In other examples of this approach, each team member is seen as the case manager. The strengths-based approach goes beyond the philosophy of identifying child and family strengths and consists of particular processes used with children and their families to secure necessary resources. Unlike approaches that focus on problem identification and solution, the strengths-based approach's focus on identifying personal abilities and family resources is central to building the plan of care. The linking of services is dictated by the mutually defined plan of care, and the implementation is executed by both the child and family as well as the case manager. When formal resources do not exist, the case manager's role is to identify and to use or create informal resources.

The various models and approaches described above outline some of the variables that differentiate among case management practices. Several authors (see Burns et al., 1995; Robinson & Toff-Bergman, 1989; Stroul, 1995) have outlined variables or factors that influence case management practices. These factors can be categorized into three broad dimensions: the organizational/system structure within which case management services are delivered; the functions performed by the case manager; and the factors relating to the implementation of case management services (see Figure 8.2). Within the organizational/system structure dimension, issues of auspices (i.e., which agency will be responsible for the provision of case management functions) and the location of case management functions (i.e., does the case management function belong within the service organization or outside it) are found. Additionally, the overarching philosophy of case management services adopted can differentiate between case management approaches and can distinguish whether the

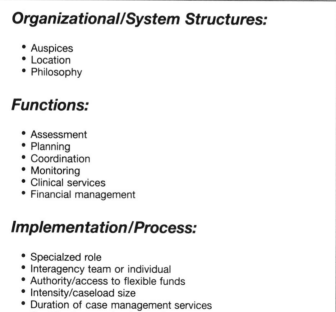

Organizational/System Structures:

- Auspices
- Location
- Philosophy

Functions:

- Assessment
- Planning
- Coordination
- Monitoring
- Clinical services
- Financial management

Implementation/Process:

- Specialzed role
- Interagency team or individual
- Authority/access to flexible funds
- Intensity/caseload size
- Duration of case management services
- Qualifications and training of case managers

Figure 8.2. Dimensions affecting the delivery of case management services.

case management and service system is family centered, individualized, and/or based on strengths.

In the dimension focusing on the functions of case management services, two additional activities are often observed. In addition to the predominant activities of assessment, planning, advocacy, monitoring, and linking of services, the inclusion of clinical services and financial management may be added to the role of the case manager. Some programs emphasize the clinical nature of the case manager's role and use the term *clinical case managers* or *therapeutic case managers*. Another influential variable affecting the delivery of case management services is whether a financial management function is included. This financial management function has generally been directed toward the goal of cost containment and is often associated with health care organizations attempting to manage the care provided to consumers to promote more efficient service delivery and to contain costs.

The factors within the implementation or process dimension examine the "how" of case management. Variables within the cluster include whether case management is seen as a specialized function or as a function added to an existing practitioner within the system of care. Whether case management services are implemented as a function of a team with a designated lead case manager or solely as a function of an individual is another variable in the implementation dimension. One of the major factors that differentiates case management practices is the authority and autonomy granted case managers in planning and implementing the intervention plan. In some approaches, case managers have the authority to control funds, usually referred to as *wraparound* or *flexible funds*, to purchase or develop services for children and families.

Another implementation factor is the intensity of case management services, the amount of time and resources devoted to each child and family; an emerging approach includes *intensive case managers* who have small caseloads, with each case requiring specialized attention as a result of the severity of problems coupled with the need for multiple services. Other implementation factors include the duration of case management services and the training and qualifications deemed necessary for case managers. Given the multitude of models presented as well as the various organizational/ system structure, process factors, and functions, there is little doubt why Burns et al. (1995) suggested that "it may be useful, for the purposes of clarifying the field and for research, to develop a schematic that describes models in terms of functions and dimensions" (p. 360).

EFFECTIVENESS AND OUTCOME RESEARCH

Studies documenting the effectiveness of case management services with adult populations are available (see Bigelow & Young, 1991; Chamberlain & Rapp, 1991; Intagliata & Baker, 1983; Rubin, 1992; Solomon, 1992). The adult literature has been useful in providing direction for the development of case management services for children and the identification of factors that affect case management services, such as size of caseloads and financing. However, these findings must be viewed with caution because the service and developmental needs of children with emotional and behavioral disorders and their families differ significantly from those of adults with mental disorders.

A number of case management programs have been developed nationwide to serve children with special needs, including those with emotional and behavioral disorders. The studies described within this chapter are organized into three categories. First, controlled studies are described that have examined the effectiveness of case management/service coordination for children who have emotional and behavioral disorders or at risk for this condition. As of 1995, six studies have been conducted within a controlled design in which participants were either randomly assigned to conditions, compared with a nontreated group, or compared with matched cases pretreatment and posttreatment to examine effectiveness. The next group of studies investigated the outcomes associated with the emerging case management model that focuses on the individualized, wraparound services approach used in North Carolina, Alaska, and Vermont. The final section of the chapter presents selected studies with a focus on case management for a variety of disability groups. Although certainly not exhaustive, this last section is included in an effort to present work that may influence and guide the continued investigation of the effectiveness of case management services for children with emotional or behavioral disorders.

Six controlled studies have examined the effects of case management within comprehensive service systems. Burns et al. (in press) and Paulson, Gratton, Stuntzer-Gibson, and Summers (1995) present research results on case management services developed within sites participating in the Robert Wood Johnson Foundation's Mental Health Services Program for Youth; and Cauce et al. (1994) and Clark et al. (1994) focus their studies on the targeted populations of homeless adolescents and children in foster care, respectively, groups comprising children and adolescents at risk for or currently identified as having emotional and behavioral disorders. The last studies, both conducted by Evans and her colleagues, examine the provision of intensive case management services to youth in New York State. One study examined pre- and postintervention comparisons for youth in the areas of community tenure and patterns of state psychiatric hospital use after receipt of case management services. The second study utilized random assignment of children referred for therapeutic foster care either to a family-centered intensive case management services group or to a family-based treatment foster care services group and compared child and family functioning for the two groups.

North Carolina

The Assessing Coordinated Care (ACC) study was carried out in conjunction with the Robert Wood Johnson Foundation's Mental Health Services Program for Youth demonstration project in the western part of North Carolina (Burns et al., in press), which included the 11 westernmost counties in the state. Although most of the essential components of a system of care were in place in this area, the capacity was not sufficient to serve the population in need of services. During the demonstration project, primary development occurred in the area of interagency relationships and system building, case management, therapeutic foster care, day treatment, and in-home services.

The ACC study was a randomized trial of the effects of case managers. Participating youth were randomly assigned to one of two conditions. In the experimental condition, youth were served by a multiagency treatment team led by a case manager. In the control condition, the treatment team was led by the youth's primary clinician from the mental health center. Burns et al. (in press) report that this study focused specifically on

> (a) activities carried out by case managers and whether these activities are similar for clinicians who were asked to fill the role of case manager; (b) differences in services resulting from the addition of a case manager to the treatment team; and (c) differences in outcomes between youths with an added case manager and those without one. (p. 7)

Essentially, this study investigated the outcomes associated with the two types of case management services models discussed earlier—that is, the clinical therapist/case manager model and the interdisciplinary team lead by a case manager model.

Baseline interviews for both parents and youth included the Child and Adolescent Psychiatric Assessment (CAPA) (Angold, Cox, Prendergast, Rutter, & Simonoff, 1992) and the Child and Adolescent Service Assessment (CASA) (Burns, Angold, Magruder-Habib, Costello, & Patrick, 1992). In addition, parents completed the Child and Adolescent Burden Assessment (CABA) (Angold et al., 1995; Patrick, Angold, Burns, & Costello, 1992) to assess family burdens associated with the youth's emotional and/or behavior problems. After the interview, the information was used to complete the Child and Adolescent Functional Assessment Scale (Hodges, 1993). This set of measures was repeated at 1 year follow-up with parents and youth. Parents also were contacted by telephone three times during the year (at 3, 6, and 9 months after the baseline interviews) to gather information on symptomatology and recent service use.

To more fully analyze issues related to case management and other service provision, two additional types of information were collected. Data were obtained from the management information systems at both participating mental health centers to document services provided over the year. Self-reports of case management activities were collected from all treatment team members using a form developed for the study, the Case Management Function Form (CMFF). This form was completed at 3-month intervals throughout the year. On this form, team members reported the number of hours spent in the previous month (either with or on behalf of a youth) and also the percentage of total time spent in various case management activities such as monitoring, advocating, and evaluation.

The ACC sample contained 167 youth, with 82 (49%) randomly assigned to the experimental group (i.e., experimental, specialized case managers) and 85 (51%) randomly assigned to the control group (i.e., primary clinicians who were placed in the role of case manager, clinician case managers). Of the youth, 97% met criteria for a DSM-III-R diagnosis or significant functional impairment (*Diagnostic and Statistical Manual of Mental Disorders*, Third Edition, Revised; American Psychiatric Association, 1987). The sample was fairly evenly divided between males and females and was predominantly white, consistent with the child population in the western region of North Carolina. Analyses of baseline data and demographic information revealed no statistical significant difference between the conditions. Additionally, refusal to participate and attrition were both low. There was an 8% refusal rate, and follow-up data for 89% ($n = 148$) of the original sample of youth were collected.

With regard to the case management activities for the two conditions, experimental case managers reported spending significantly more time with or on behalf of their clients. They also spent their time in a way that differed significantly from the clinical case managers. Experimental case managers spent more time on the core functions of case management: outreach; assessment of strengths, needs, and resources; service planning and monitoring; linking, referral, and advocacy; and crisis intervention.

Another area of investigation within the study was whether the two case management approaches were associated with differences in the provision of other types of mental health services. Results revealed that youth with experimental case managers remained in the program longer, received a richer array of services during the final months of the intervention, and were more likely to receive community-based (as opposed to out-of-community) services. Youth in the experimental group also were less likely to have received inpatient services during follow-up than were youth in the control group.

Investigations of other family and individual outcomes revealed that the youth and their families in both conditions improved over the course of the year. Overall improvements were seen in functional status as measured by Child and Adolescent Functional Assessment Scale (CAFAS) scores and incapacity scores from the CAPA, number of symptoms, and family burden; however, there were no significant differences in improvement between the two groups. There was a significant difference in that the parents of youth in the experimental group reported greater satisfaction with the mental health center services, and the same youth showed less impairment due to alcohol consumption.

Multnomah County, Oregon

The Partners' Project, operating in the vicinity surrounding Portland, was also a demonstration site of the Robert Wood Johnson Foundation's Mental Health Services Program for Youth. This project used pooled funding between multiple agencies to build community-based services and created a multiagency board to coordinate service planning and delivery (Paulson et al., 1995). The focus of the evaluation was to study the effectiveness of case management and flexible funding on service processes and outcomes for children with serious emotional disorders and their families. From its inception in August 1990 through June 1994, 361 youth and families have been served. To be eligible for services, youth had to be between the ages of 5 and 18, have involvement in two or more public agencies to address functional impairment, and be at risk of a restrictive, out-of-home placement.

Initial results on characteristics of the youth served by the Partners' Project ($n = 115$) revealed that the majority were male (64%), were Caucasian (77%), and had an average age of a little over 12 years. Furthermore, the majority of youth had experienced an out-of-home placement (54%), and 42% were in the custody of the state of Oregon. On a measure of psychopathology, the Child Behavior Checklist (CBCL) (Achenbach & Edelbrock, 1983), more than three quarters of the youth scored within the clinical range on the Total Problem, Internalizing, and Externalizing scales (93%, 77%, and 87%, respectively).

An initial analysis of data collected 12 months post-enrollment revealed that families in the Partner's Project experienced greater individualization, coordination, and comprehensiveness in service delivery as compared with youth receiving services "as usual" ($n = 117$). Both youth and caregivers in the project reported greater satisfaction and greater empowerment than the comparison group, and project youth scored significantly better than the comparison youth on measures of social competence. The two groups did not differ, however, on measures of psychopathology or in the level of restrictiveness of service delivery at the 12-month assessment. These results must be viewed with caution because the youth in the comparison group, who were youth identified and served by the educational system, were significantly less impaired (as measured by the CBCL) than the youth participating in the project.

Continued investigations are planned for the evaluation of this project. These include longitudinal analyses of service coordination and related outcomes, an analysis of outcomes for youth who had case managers with access to flexible funds compared with a group of youth who had case managers without this option, and analyses of the costs associated with providing case management services with flexible funding.

Washington State

An evaluation of an innovative, intensive mental health case management program for homeless adolescents in Seattle, Washington, has been undertaken by Cauce and her colleagues (Cauce et al., 1994). This innovative program differs from services as usual in that caseload size is limited to 12 youth, the amount of supervision and the resources made available to case managers is increased, and the educational level of case managers is higher than that of case managers providing services as usual. An analysis of data gathered on youth randomly assigned to the innovative case management ($n = 55$) versus the regular case management program ($n = 60$) collected during the first 3 months of the program indicated that for self-reported levels of aggression, general externalizing behavior, and satisfaction with quality of life, there was a trend for youth assigned to the innovative program to improve more than youth receiving regular case management services.

Florida

Clark et al. (1994) reported the preliminary findings of the Fostering Individualized Assistance Program (FIAP) study, which involved a comparison of children in foster care randomly assigned to the FIAP program (FIAP group) or to a group that received standard-practice (SP) foster care services (SP group). The FIAP program sought to stabilize foster care placement and to develop viable permanency plans as well as to improve the behavioral and emotional adjustment of youth participating in the program. Family specialists, who served as clinical case managers and home-based counselors, implemented the four intervention components of strengths-based assessment, life-domain planning, clinical case management, and follow-up supports and services (see Clark et al., 1994, for a description of the FIAP model).

Child outcome data were collected across a number of domains and included measures of behavioral and emotional adjustment, out-of-home placement information, and detention/jail and felony records. Preliminary data ($N = 132$) suggested the following results. 1) Results of the CBCL (Achenbach, 1991a) indicated that children in the FIAP group improved significantly more from admission to 18 months later on the withdrawn and attention problem subscales than did children in the SP group. Across all problem subscales, the FIAP group evidenced lower pathology scores than did the SP group. 2) No significant differences were noted between the groups on the Youth Self Report Scale (YSR; Achenbach,

1991b). 3) For a limited number of youth in the sample in permanency placements (i.e., biological, adoptive, or relative home) at 18 months after entrance into the study, the results indicated greater emotional adjustment for the FIAP subsample based on the caregivers' perspective and greater behavioral adjustment for the FIAP subsample based on the youths' perspective in contrast with the SP subsample. 4) Finally, those in the FIAP group were found to be less likely to run away, engage in serious criminal activity, or be jailed, although both groups showed improvement over the first 18 months of the study.

New York State

Evans, Banks, et al. (1994) described New York State's Intensive Case Management Program for Children and Youth (CYICM), best described as an Expanded Broker Model (see Robinson, 1991, for a description of this model). The case management program was an intensive, client-centered linkage and advocacy-focused model implemented in 42 counties in the state. Case managers had small caseloads (10:1) and provided assessment, planning, linking, and advocacy services. The primary goal of CYICM was to place children with serious emotional and behavioral disorders in the least restrictive environment appropriate to their needs.

Data on the effectiveness of case management in preventing hospitalization and increasing community tenure are presented here. Data were gathered from a Client Description Form and the Department of Mental Hygiene Information System that tracked the movement of all persons within the state psychiatric hospital system. Two analytic techniques were used to assess effectiveness. A preenrollment/postenrollment matched case community tenure analysis was conducted to examine whether length of stay in the community between admissions to the state psychiatric hospital after CYICM enrollment was significantly longer than the time observed between hospital stays for the same cases in the preenrollment period. Results of an analysis of a sample of 87 children revealed that postenrollment time intervals between admissions were longer after CYICM (average of 574 days) than prior to this service (average of 122 days).

An analysis of patterns of state psychiatric hospital utilization was also conducted. This analysis involved a preintervention/postintervention comparison of utilization levels and was conducted to determine whether the observed changes in inpatient utilization were due to enrollment in CYICM. Using a sample of 526 children, results revealed that system utilization shifted to a lower level after CYICM enrollment. Overall, the data suggested that CYICM was associated with fewer hospitalizations, fewer hospital days, and more days spent in the community after enrollment as compared with pre-CYICM enrollment of children with serious emotional and behavioral disorders.

Evans, Armstrong, et al. (1994) presented the preliminary findings of another study of New York's intensive case management model for children and youth with serious emotional and behavioral disorders. Under controlled experimental conditions, children referred for therapeutic foster care in three rural New York counties were randomly assigned to groups receiving Family-Centered Intensive Case Management (FCICM) services or Family-Based Treatment (FBT) foster care services. FCICM was a community-based program designed to empower and support the families of children with serious emotional and behavioral disorders. Utilizing a case manager and parent advocate, the FCICM intervention included respite services, flexible service money, parent support groups, and parent skills training. FBT was New York's treatment foster care program designed to provide the least restrictive placement for children with serious emotional and behavioral disorders who required treatment in an out-of-home setting. The program provided training, support, and respite to professional families and allowed the child to be cared for in a family-based setting. When possible, children were reunited with the biological family after treatment goals were achieved.

Assessments of child and family functioning were conducted at referral, every 6 months during treatment, and at 6 months postdischarge. Preliminary 6-month data were available for 22 children and families. Data at 6 months focused on measures of family functioning, child symptomatology, and changes in service needs. For the entire group, as well as by program type, the level of unmet need either decreased or remained unchanged, except in the area of recreation. Across interventions, the greatest decreases in service needs were in the areas of education and mental health. Whereas all children in the FCICM group were in need of recreational services at admission and at 6 months follow-up, there was a decrease in need from admission to 6 months for 45% of the children in the FBT group.

The Parent Skills Index (Magura & Moses, 1986) was utilized as a measure of family functioning. For parents in both the FBT and FCICM groups, there was a slight but positive change on four of the six scales from admission to 6 months (Motivation to Solve Problems, Approval of Children, Consistency of Discipline, and Teaching/Stimulation of Children). There was a slight decrease on the Recognition of Problems and Acceptance/Affection for Children scales. In a comparison of parents in the FBT and FCICM groups, FBT natural parents improved or maintained their scores on all six scales from admission to 6 months. Results for the FCICM parents were mixed. Scores increased on three scales and decreased on the other three scales. Parents in the FCICM group had better scores than did parents in the FBT group on the Consistency of Discipline and the Approval of Children scales.

Scores on the Child and Adolescent Functional Assessment Scales (Hodges, 1993) were significantly improved in the areas of Role Performance and Moods/Emotions. Furthermore, the mean number of problem behaviors and symptoms as measured by the CBCL (Achenbach, 1991a) decreased for both groups between admission ($\overline{X}$ = 5.4) and 6-month follow-up ($\overline{X}$ = 3.6) (Mary Evans, personal communication, February 14, 1994). The authors stated that the lack of dramatic change or differences in outcomes across conditions was expected because findings are based on 6-month outcomes only. Greater differences between the two conditions are expected after analysis of long-term data.

INDIVIDUALIZED SERVICES MODEL
Another important characteristic within a system of care is the principle of individualized care. Based on a thorough as-

sessment of the child and the family, individualized programs are custom designed to meet the individual needs of each child and his or her family (Burns & Friedman, 1990). Individualized care has been characterized by the key elements of case management/case coordination, wraparound services, flexible funding and services, interagency collaboration (Katz-Leavy et al., 1992), unconditional care, least restrictive care, and child- and family-centered care (Burchard & Clarke, 1990).

Although the concept of individualized care was one of the original Child and Adolescent Service System Program (CASSP) values (Stroul & Friedman, 1986), it has taken a considerable period of time for this concept to be incorporated into actual practice (Research and Training Center for Children's Mental Health, 1988). Brief descriptions and available outcome data of approaches to the delivery of individualized services to children with serious emotional and behavioral disorders and their families are provided here. For a full description of programs using an individualized services approach, an excellent monograph on this topic is *Individualized Services in a System of Care* (see Katz-Leavy et al., 1992).

North Carolina

One of the first systems of care to incorporate the concept of individualized care was developed in North Carolina (Behar, 1985). In response to a lawsuit, the state of North Carolina developed the Willie M. Program, a well-funded full range of community-based services for children and adolescents who had serious emotional, neurological, or mental disorders and were violent or assaultive.

In an evaluation of the Willie M. Program, Weisz, Walter, Weiss, Fernandez, and Mikov (1990) conducted a pretest/posttest comparison of time of first arrest for two groups of individuals who had emotional disturbances and were violent and assaultive. The short-certification group ($n = 21$) was composed of individuals who had received services through the Willie M. Program for fewer than 3 months, whereas individuals in the long-certification group ($n = 147$) had received services for more than 1 year. Groups were comparable on demographic characteristics, problem behavior histories, IQ, diagnosis, and age at earliest antisocial act.

The results of a survival analysis revealed that the long-certification group showed a somewhat more favorable survival curve than did the short-certification group; however, this difference did not reach statistical significance. Thus, these findings do not appear to provide strong support for the reduction of risk of later arrest among violent and assaultive youth after participation in the Willie M. Program. The authors suggested a number of reasons for these findings. Arrest data may not serve as the most sensitive indicator of success for the program. Furthermore, no true control group exists for the comparison of individuals receiving services through the Willie M. Program. These findings are based on data gathered during the early years of the program and may not reflect the current functioning and therefore current effectiveness of the program.

Alaska Youth Initiative (AYI)

AYI represents one of the most comprehensive examples of individualized care available to date (Burchard & Clarke, 1990). The Alaska Youth Initiative, adapted from the Kaleidoscope program in Chicago, used individualized care to return children with severe behavioral and emotional disorders from out-of-state, residential programs. The demonstration project, conducted from 1986 to 1991, was created to provide individualized, community-based, wraparound services to children with serious emotional and behavioral disorders. Burchard, Burchard, Sewell, and VanDenBerg (1993) reported the results of a qualitative case study evaluation of 10 youth deemed to be among the most difficult-to-serve children and youth in Alaska; that is, children and youth for whom all available alternatives to long-term residential treatment had failed. Qualitative data were gathered through record reviews and structured interviews with service providers, families, and youth.

A qualitative analysis of the cases revealed that for 9 of the 10 cases, AYI served as a successful alternative to long-term residential treatment. For 6 of the 10 cases, children and youth were successfully reintegrated and socialized in their own or a nearby community after discharge from restrictive residential placement. During their participation in AYI, 9 youth were assisted in becoming more independent and responsible, socially appropriate, and acceptable to themselves and their communities.

At the time of the study, 9 youth had lived in open settings in their respective communities from 1 to 3 years. These settings included the home of the parents, apartments in the community, supervised apartments, and therapeutic foster care. Of the 8 older youth, 5 had been discharged from AYI and were living in the community. In interviews conducted at 6 months postdischarge, 4 of the 8 older youth reported that they were confident of their ability to continue to live unsupervised in the community. The remaining 5 children and youth were still receiving active treatment through AYI. Two of the children were in specialized foster homes and general school placements. The remaining 3 had returned from restrictive, lengthy institutional placements and had received community-based services for 3–12 months.

With regard to educational outcomes, 3 of the children who were in school at the time of the evaluation had been reintegrated successfully into mainstream schools and classes for most or all of their course work, and two of the three children were receiving high marks on a consistent basis. Five of the older youth had either successfully graduated from high school or had obtained a general equivalency diploma (GED). Based on this qualitative evaluation, it appears that the provision of individualized care through the AYI model proved effective in serving as an alternative to restrictive residential treatment for a sample of the most challenging youth in Alaska.

Vermont

Since the 1980s, Vermont has been progressively building a statewide comprehensive system of care. At the core of this system is an individualized service approach that emphasizes child- and family-centered treatment, individually tailored and flexible services provided in the least restrictive setting, flexible funding, and interagency collaboration. Individualized services are provided through a statewide therapeutic case management system (Yoe, Bruns, & Burchard, 1995).

Clarke, Schaefer, Burchard, and Welkowitz (1992) reported the findings of an evaluation of Project Wraparound, a 3-year demonstration project in which individualized care was used to prevent the placement of children in out-of-home settings. Project Wraparound was a community-based individualized treatment program in Vermont that provided intensive home- and school-based services to children and youth with severely maladjusted behavior and their families.

The purpose of the evaluation was to determine whether children who received wraparound services experienced a decrease in behavioral symptomatology in home and school settings as indicated by measures of child and family adjustment. The sample used in the analysis of home data comprised 19 families and their children, and an additional 12 children were included in the analysis of school data.

Measures of child adjustment included the Child Behavior Checklist (CBCL; Achenbach & Edelbrock, 1983), the Teacher Report Form (TRF; Achenbach & Edelbrock, 1986), the Self-Control Rating Scale (SCRS; Kendall & Wilcox, 1979), and the Connors Hyperkinesis Index (CHI; Goyette, Connors, & Ulrich, 1978). Measures of home environment included the Child Well-Being Scales (CWBS; Magura & Moses, 1986). Results of child adjustment measures indicated a significant improvement in child behavioral adjustment during the 6-month intensive home intervention period, with increased improvement over the course of the year. Improvements in behavior were not achieved in the school setting. Results of the CWBS (home environment) indicated a highly significant positive change on Composite and Parental Disposition scores; however, results for the Household Adequacy and Child Performance Subscales were not significant. Thus, Project Wraparound appears to have been effective in the improvement of child and family functioning in the home setting; however, there was no evidence of behavioral improvements in the school setting. The authors suggested a number of possible explanations for these findings (e.g., schools provided inadequate psychological services, schools were not receptive to the practice of mainstreaming children with serious emotional and behavioral disorders, mainstreaming may not be the most effective method for improving the behavior of some children with serious emotional disorders). Another explanation for these findings was the use of a small sample size.

Rosen et al. (1994) examined client satisfaction as an outcome for youth (N = 20) who received community-based, wraparound services in Vermont. Youth were queried about their satisfaction with services, their sense of involvement, and their feelings of unconditional care. (Unconditional care is defined as the "youth's sense that his or her caretakers would remain stable regardless of what happened" [Rosen, Heckman, Carro, & Burchard, 1994, p. 55].) Results found that a sense of involvement and the perception of unconditional care were strongly associated with satisfaction with services and service providers. Neither satisfaction nor involvement was associated with the severity of the youth's behavior. The perception of unconditional care had a strong, negative association with the severity of the youths' behaviors. The authors concluded that, although the relationship between satisfaction and behavioral adjustment remains equivocal, the youths' perceptions of unconditional care does appear to contribute to behavioral adjustment.

In an additional study on the outcomes of youth involved in the individualized services program in Vermont, Yoe et al. (1995) investigated the level of restrictiveness in both living arrangements and educational placements for 40 youth upon entry and again 12 months after entry into the program. Upon entry, the majority of youth (78%) were in the custody of the child welfare system and were either referred from or being referred to residential treatment placements. Overall, at the end of 12 months, youth tended to move to less restrictive living and educational environments, with 90% of the youth successfully maintained in the community over the 12-month period.

In a study to document the cost of Vermont's individualized services approach, Tighe and Brooks (1995) compared the 12-month cost incurred by 40 youth within the New Directions Program, a site participating in the Robert Wood Johnson Foundation's Mental Health Initiative for Youth Program, with the costs incurred by 26 youth being served in out-of-state residential treatment facilities. Of the total costs for the New Directions Program, 40% were living-related expenses such as foster care, professional roommates, and independent living expenses. Education-related expenses comprised approximately 26% of the total costs, and case management made up another 22%. The remaining costs were incurred for services such as respite, social skills training, therapy, and emergency services.

The total cost of individualized services, on average, was $4,036 a month or $48,432 a year for each child. In comparison, the average cost for the out-of-state, residential treatment programs was $4,893 a month or $58,716 a year for each child. Multiple agencies and systems provided funding to cover costs of the New Directions Program, with the educational system providing 34% of the total costs, federal funding providing 30% under Title IV-E and Title XIX of the Social Security Act, child welfare providing 24%, mental health providing 10% of the total costs, and 2% from other sources.

CASE MANAGEMENT FOR OTHER POPULATIONS OF CHILDREN

Children with Developmental Disabilities

Singer, Irvin, Irvine, Hawkins, and Cooley (1989) conducted a study of the families of children with significant developmental disabilities. Families were randomly assigned to one of two groups: 1) *modest service*, which consisted of the provision of respite care and case management services; or 2) *intensive service*, which consisted of stress management, parenting skills training, support groups, and community-based respite care. A significantly greater number of parents in the intensive services group achieved clinically significant improvement on measures of anxiety and depression. These findings suggested that comprehensive services provided directly to families was more effective than the provision of case management and respite services alone.

Children at Risk for Dropping Out

Stowitschek and Smith (1990) described the development and implementation of an interprofessional case management model (C-STARS) for dropout prevention programming in school/community sites in Washington State. The model comprised four components: 1) direction and development of case management services; 2) generic case management functions, which included the identification and assessment of students, advocacy efforts, development of a service plan, brokering of services, implementation of a service plan, mentoring, and evaluation and tracking; 3) special implementation considerations pertaining to program quality, equity, and comprehensiveness; and 4) assistance of a university interdisciplinary team that provided technical guidance, training, and other support services.

Nine school/community sites participated in the project. First-year results of a formative evaluation of the C-STARS case management model revealed that sites reported that at least 85% of the generic elements of interprofessional case management had been implemented for at-risk students. Individual service plans had been completed for a total of 87 students. *All* service goals had been attained for 35% of these students, and at least one service goal had been attained for 68%. Moderate changes were reported for three targeted risk measures: the percentage of students whose absences exceeded 10 or more days per semester decreased from 73% to 40%; the number of students earning one or more unacceptable grades decreased from 82% to 54%; and the percentage of students receiving one or more days of poor conduct reports decreased from 95% to 71%. The most significant outcomes reported by case managers were graduation of students, increased participation in school, and higher levels of family involvement.

Homeless Youth

Stoep and Blanchard (1992) reported the findings of the evaluation of a mental health case management service program for homeless youth in Seattle, Washington. Case management services were delivered to homeless youth through a licensed mental health agency for 9 months. The multiservice center provided meals, recreation, counseling, health screening, a school program, and referrals to local agencies for homeless and street youth who had not been served successfully by traditional mental health services. An attempt was made to increase the clients' opportunities to return to their home by offering services to the family. Case plans were developed collaboratively by an interdisciplinary treatment team, the youth, and the family. Treatment outcomes for two groups were based on data gathered from screening/intake forms, service logs, and interviews with case managers. The client group (n = 28) was composed of youth who were provided with a mental health case manager and received services, and the contact group (n = 48) included youth who had some contact with mental health case managers but did not complete the intake process. For the total of 76 youth who had contact with case managers during the 17-month project (October 1990–February 1992), desirable outcomes were achieved in the six areas assessed: 11 youth (14%) were returned to their local community, 17 (22%) were linked with resources to work with parents, and 16 (21%) were assisted in reentering entitlement or treatment programs. A total of 19 youth (25%) were assisted in gaining placement in a house or shelter, 10 youth (13%) were helped to obtain job training, and 8 (10%) received a GED.

A comparison of the two groups revealed that a higher percentage of youth in the client group achieved the desired treatment outcomes as compared with youth in the contact group. For the client group, over 32% achieved the outcomes of working with parents, securing shelter, and obtaining entitlement, whereas a smaller percentage of those in the contact group achieved these same outcomes (17%, 21%, and 15%, respectively). About 14% of the youth in the client group obtained a GED, whereas approximately 8% did so in the contact group. Greater than 20% of those in the client group received job training, as compared with about 8% of the contact group.

At-Risk Youth

The SUCCESS program, implemented in the Des Moines (Iowa) public school system, was developed to provide case management services to children and families at risk of not achieving the goals of their educational programs or thriving in their families and/or communities. Community resources were integrated within the school system through the use of family resource centers. The SUCCESS program was based on the provision of case management services to targeted families; the location of human services staff in the schools; and the provision of referral and intensive follow-up services.

Findings are derived from the first formal evaluation of services and outcomes based on 270 children and youth. According to the planning/evaluation report for 1990–1991 (Des Moines [Iowa] Public Schools, 1991), students receiving case management services made progress in the areas of attendance, grade point averages, reduced suspensions, reenrollment of dropouts, participation in extracurricular activities, and family environments. Furthermore, reactions from parents and students were positive, and services were perceived as helpful. A more rigorous evaluation of program outcomes is planned.

Children with Developmental Disabilities and Health Problems

Marcenko and Smith (1992) reported the findings of a study that examined the impact of a family-centered case management approach for the families of children with both a developmental disability and an ongoing health condition. Mental retardation and cerebral palsy were the most frequent developmental disabilities, and ongoing health conditions varied among mucopolysaccharidosis, diaphragmatic hernia, and bronchial pulmonary dysplasia. A family-centered case management program focuses on the "family as a constant in the child's life and thus emphasizes parent/professional collaboration, and the responsiveness of the service system to family needs" (Marcenko & Smith, 1992, p. 90). Programs were based on a services management model with the goal of providing services to increase the potential of the person with a disability and his or her family in the areas of independence, productivity, and community integration. Strategies implemented to meet this goal included outreach, coordination, brokering, monitoring, advocating, training, and interdisciplinary team planning. Primary activities of project staff included working with parents in groups, arranging for support services, obtaining financial assistance for services, counseling, and performing administrative tasks. Service plans were developed in collaboration with the family, social workers, school personnel, and medical professionals. Interventions were conducted with families in their homes, the hospital, schools, and at the social service agency. Data ($N = 32$ families) were gathered during the first month of participation in the project and approximately 1 year later. Instruments included a semistructured questionnaire designed to evaluate program impact and an intake instrument that gathered information on sociodemographics, service utilization and satisfaction, family stress and coping, and maternal life satisfaction.

The assessment of the impact of the case management program was based largely on service needs assessment and changes in service use. The most significant increases in service use were in the areas of regular respite care and home nursing. Small increases also were noted in the frequency with which families used education services, child care training, transportation to school, and routine medical services. Families continued to indicate a high level of need for recreational activities, life planning services, legal services, regular child care, and speech therapy.

Data regarding program effectiveness were gathered by asking mothers to identify the ways in which they had benefitted from services provided by project staff. Mothers noted the following benefits: greater access to services, assistance with the financing of services, opportunities to become involved with and to receive emotional support from other families and staff, information about caring for their child, and the development of advocacy skills. Mean ratings of maternal satisfaction with current life situation, as measured on a 10-point Likert scale, revealed a statistically significant increase from intake (5.39) to follow-up (6.25). A 5-point Likert scale was used to measure the coping ability of siblings without disabilities. Findings revealed a nonsignificant but slight decrease in the mean ratings of coping skills of siblings without disabilities between intake (2.41) and follow-up (2.77). Thus, the findings indicated that family-centered case management services were beneficial to families, particularly in the areas of gaining access to existing services and increasing maternal life satisfaction. It should be noted, however, that no control group was used. Thus, it is not known if the same gains would have been experienced in the absence of case management services.

Children at Risk for Substance Abuse

Muller et al. (1992) reported the results of a demonstration project designed to develop and investigate innovative interventions for children at high risk for substance abuse disorders in Alabama. Participants in the project consisted of 171 youth and their families who met at least 2 of 17 risk factors related to substance abuse. Participants were placed in one of two intervention groups: Case Management Intervention ($n = 112$) or Home-Based Intervention plus Case Management Follow-up Services ($n = 59$). Those who were at imminent risk for removal from the home were targeted for the more intensive home-based intervention group. Children placed in the Home-Based Intervention plus Case Management Follow-up group received 3 months of home-based intervention followed by 1 year of case management follow-up services. A two-member team worked with families in their homes for about two 2-hour sessions on a weekly basis throughout the 3-month intervention period. Services were family focused and ecologically based and included outreach services, crisis intervention services, family training and counseling, modeling, and individualized goal contracting. During follow-up, case managers functioned in the areas of linking families to services, advocacy, information dissemination, referral, and monitoring. Those in the Case Management Intervention group received 15 months of case management services only. The duties of the case manager consisted of outreach, service planning, service linking, advocacy, information dissemination, referral, and monitoring.

At pretest and posttest, children and their families were administered a battery of instruments to measure service needs and functioning. Assessment instruments included the Service Utilization and Needs Assessment Instrument, which measured the need for socialization/recreation, education, daily living skills training, transportation, financial, medical, mental health, and housing services. The Environmental Deprivation Scale was administered to assess the client's level of adaptive functioning in the following areas: educational/ school activities, leisure time activities, interpersonal interactions, and self-management behaviors. The Maladaptive Behavior Record was used to identify specific maladaptive behaviors. Parenting skills and other adaptive parent characteristics were assessed for both the mother and father via the Parent Input Index. The Drug Evaluation Scale and the Alcohol Evaluation Scale were used to determine alcohol and drug use for each client. At baseline, median total scores on all measures were similar across the groups for both interventions and were indicative of severe maladaptation on all assessment instruments. Furthermore, baseline outcome measures were similar for both groups.

Results revealed two major findings. First, those families and children who had maintained a longer relationship with service providers fared better in all areas of functioning. Furthermore, families who refused to participate or dropped out of the intervention after receiving minimal participation experienced fewer improvements in functioning and in fact exhibited some declines in functioning over time.

A second significant finding revealed that the group receiving Home-Based Intervention plus Case Management Follow-up Services showed greater improvement in all areas of functioning, with the exception of alcohol and drug abuse, as compared with the Case Management Intervention group. For both intervention groups, the greatest improvements were in the areas of meeting needs for community services and increasing service utilization. Thus, these results suggested that both the Case Management Intervention and Home-Based Intervention plus Case Management Follow-up Services were effective interventions for families with youth at high risk for substance abuse. However, the limited effect of these interventions on alcohol and drug abuse suggested that these particular behaviors may be the most resistant and may be the last to change.

Evans, Dollard, and McNulty (1992) described the characteristics of youth with and without substance abuse being served in New York State's CYICM and their use of inpatient services before and after enrollment in CYICM. As described in the previous section of this chapter, the case management program in New York was a client-centered linkage and advocacy-focused model of case management implemented in 42 counties across the state. Case managers had a small caseload (10:1), and services were delivered in natural settings.

A total of 664 adolescents were served by CYICM, and 145 (22%) of this total number were defined as substance abusers. Criteria for classification as a substance abuser included a history of alcohol or substance abuse treatment, a DSM-III-R alcohol or drug diagnosis, the display of symptoms of alcohol or drug abuse upon enrollment in CYICM, or a referral for alcohol or substance abuse treatment upon discharge from CYICM. For the purposes of this review, only results pertaining to the effects of CYICM in reducing residential placement are presented (see Evans et al., 1992, for a review of the characteristics of this population). To measure the effectiveness of CYICM in the prevention of unnecessary restrictive placement, change in the living situation of youth between admission and discharge was assessed. Environments were rank-ordered based on level of restrictiveness, with independent living rated as least restrictive and institutional living rated as most restrictive. For both the substance-abusing and non–substance-abusing groups, living situation at discharge from CYICM was significantly different from the living situation at admission. For the group of substance abusers ($n = 52$), 73% had no change in living situation between admission and discharge, 4% moved to a less restrictive placement, and 23% moved to a more restrictive placement setting. Of the non–substance-abusing group ($n = 140$), 68% had no change between admission and discharge, 8% moved to a less restrictive setting, and 24% moved to a more restrictive placement.

A reduction in the number of hospital admissions and days spent in inpatient settings was used as another measure of the effectiveness of preventing unnecessary restrictive placement. Data for the 12 months preceding admission to CYICM and the 12 months following admission to CYICM were analyzed for a total of 157 youth. No significant differences were noted in the average number of state inpatient admissions between the groups in either the 12 months preceding or following admission to CYICM. However, within-group comparisons of the pre- and postenrollment periods revealed that the average number of admissions was significantly higher in the preadmission period for both groups. With regard to the number of days spent in inpatient settings, a within-group comparison of the pre- and postenrollment periods indicated that the average number of days spent in state hospitals was significantly higher in the preenrollment period for both groups. No significant difference was noted between the two groups in postadmission length of stay (27 vs. 14 days); however, non–substance abusers spent significantly more days on average in state hospitals during the preenrollment period (82 vs. 53 days). Further analysis revealed no significant difference between the groups in the reduction of average inpatient days from pre- to postenrollment periods. Thus, the CYICM intervention was not more effective for one group than for the other in reducing the number of days spent in the hospital in the postadmission period. The authors concluded that the CYICM intervention was associated with a decrease in hospital admissions and total number of days spent in inpatient settings after admission to CYICM for all youth, including those with substance abuse problems. Results should be viewed with caution due to the absence of a comparison group.

CONCLUSIONS AND FUTURE RESEARCH NEEDS

The provision of case management services is a rapidly developing effort aimed at meeting the complex and multidimensional needs of children with special needs and their families. The primary role of the case manager is to ensure that services are delivered in an effective and efficient manner. A number of case management models exist. Approaches range from those in which the case manager acts as a broker with the primary responsibility of making arrangements for clients to receive services to a full-support model in which the case manager provides specific clinical tasks in addition to the brokering of services.

Few well-controlled studies of case management exist for the children's mental health field (Burns et al., 1995). This paucity of research stems from two primary factors: 1) the difficulty in determining separate contribution of case management services to the overall effectiveness of a continuum of care, and 2) the recency of the provision of case management services to children with serious emotional problems and their families. Despite these factors, six controlled studies have been conducted to determine the effectiveness of case management services for children with serious emotional and behavioral disorders and their families.

Summary

Two studies present research results on case management services developed within sites participating in the Robert Wood Johnson Foundation's Mental Health Services Program for Youth. The study by Burns et al. (in press) investigated the outcomes associated between two types of case management services: the clinical therapist/case manager model and the interdisciplinary team lead by a case manager model. Results revealed that experimental case managers reported spending significantly more time with or on behalf of their clients and spent more time on the core functions of case management. Youth with experimental case managers remained in the program for a longer period of time, received a richer array of services during the final months of the intervention, and were more likely to receive community-based (as opposed to out-of-community) services. Youth in the experimental group were less likely to have received inpatient services during follow-up than were youth in the control group. Investigations of other family and individual outcomes revealed that the youth and their families in both conditions improved over the course of the year. Furthermore, parents of youth in the experimental group reported greater satisfaction with the mental health center services, and the same youth showed less impairment due to alcohol consumption.

Initial findings for the Partners' Project in Portland, Oregon (Paulson et al.,1995), indicated that, compared with families receiving services "as usual," those families participating in the project reported greater individualization, coordination, and comprehensiveness in service delivery at 12 months postenrollment. Furthermore, greater satisfaction and sense of empowerment were reported by both youth and caregivers in the project compared with the comparison group, and youth participating in the project scored significantly higher on measures of social competence than did youth in the comparison group. The groups did not differ, however, on measures of psychopathology or level of restrictiveness of service delivery at the 12-month assessment. The authors indicate that these results must be viewed with caution because youth in the comparison group were significantly less impaired than were youth participating in the project.

Preliminary results of the studies by Cauce et al. (1994) and Clark et al. (1994), which focused on the targeted populations of homeless adolescents and children in foster care, revealed generally positive results for youth receiving case management services as compared with those receiving standard practice. For the targeted population of homeless youth, an analysis of data gathered on youth randomly assigned to the innovative case management versus regular case management program collected during the first 3 months of the program indicated that, for self-reported levels of aggression, general externalizing behavior, and satisfaction with quality of life, there was a trend for youths assigned to the innovative program to improve more than youth receiving regular case management services (Cauce et al., 1994). Findings for the study targeting youth in foster care revealed that children in the FIAP group improved significantly more from admission to 18 months later on the withdrawn and attention problem subscales than did the children in the standard practice group and evidenced lower pathology scores across all subscales. No significant differences were noted between the groups on the Youth Self Report Scale. For a limited number of youth in permanency placements at 18 months after entrance into the study, the results indicated greater emotional and behavioral adjustment for the FIAP subsample in contrast with the standard practice subsample. Furthermore, the FIAP group was found to be less likely to run away, engage in serious criminal activity, or be jailed, although both groups showed improvement over the first 18 months of the study.

The last studies, both conducted by Evans and her colleagues, examined the provision of intensive case management services to youth in New York State. In the first study,
Evans, Banks, et al. (1994) revealed that the provision of
case management services was associated with fewer hospitalizations, fewer hospital days, and more days spent in
the community. The second study, conducted by Evans,
Armstrong, et al. (1994), examined the effectiveness of two intensive community-based programs for children with serious emotional and behavioral disorders and their families:
Family-Centered Intensive Case Management services and
Family-Based Treatment Foster Care services. Preliminary 6-month data found no dramatic change or differences
across the two conditions in the areas of service needs,
family functioning, and child symptomatology. Greater differences are expected when long-term data are analyzed.

The principle of individualized care calls for the delivery
of services that meet the unique needs and potentials of each
individual child and family. As was true for the area of case
management, little research has been conducted to examine
the effectiveness of individualized care. This perhaps results
from the great variability in the types of problem behavior
exhibited by the children served and, consequently, from the
fact that no two children receive the same array of services.

Three programs that have incorporated the principle of
individualized care for children and youth with serious emotional disorders were reviewed. The results of data examining
the effectiveness of individualized care were mixed. The evaluation of the Willie M. Program in the state of North Carolina
did not provide strong support for the reduction of risk of
later arrest among violent and assaultive youth after participation in the program. In contrast, a qualitative analysis of
10 youth who participated in the Alaska Youth Initiative revealed that the provision of individualized care through the
AYI model was effective in serving as an alternative to restrictive residential treatment for a sample of the most challenging youth in Alaska. A number of studies have evaluated
the effectiveness of Project Wraparound in Vermont. One
study indicated the effectiveness of the program in improving child and family functioning in the home setting; how-

ever, behavioral improvements did not generalize to the school setting (Clarke et al., 1992). Rosen et al. (1994) examined client satisfaction as an outcome for youth ($N = 20$) who received community-based, wraparound services in Vermont and found that the relationship between satisfaction and behavioral adjustment was equivocal; however, the authors concluded that the youth's perceptions of unconditional care did appear to contribute to behavioral adjustment. Yoe et al. (1995) investigated the level of restrictiveness in living arrangements and educational placements for 40 youth upon entry and again 12 months after entry into the program. Overall, at the end of 12 months, youth tended to move to less restrictive living and educational environments, with 90% of the youth successfully maintained in the community over the 12-month period. An average cost of $4,036 per month for each child receiving individualized services was found (Tighe & Brooks, 1995).

Studies that examined the efficacy of case management services for children with special needs other than serious emotional problems were reviewed. The studies contained in the present chapter included a variety of populations, such as children with developmental disabilities and ongoing health conditions, homeless children and youth, at-risk children and youth, and youth with substance abuse problems. The results of these studies revealed generally positive outcomes across a variety of domains for those receiving case management services.

Conclusions

Case management services is one of the newer and more complex approaches for working with children and families. In this section, six studies designed to evaluate the effectiveness of case management services were reviewed. Target populations varied within these studies, as did the research designs and the models of case management under investigation. Consequently, the research base is still too limited to allow any definitive conclusion as to the effectiveness of this service.

Two studies, Clark et al. (1994) and Paulson et al. (1995), compared youth receiving case management services with youth who did not receive this service. Whereas Paulson and his colleagues (1995) found increased service coordination and integration for the case management group, no differences between groups in measures of psychopathology were found. Conversely, Clark et al. (1994) found symptom reduction in a few areas; however, he did not examine outcomes in terms of service integration and coordination.

Two other studies, Burns et al. (in press) and Cauce et al. (1994), examined outcomes associated with different models of case management services. Cauce's initial analysis found some positive differences in psychological and social adjustment for youth assigned to an intensive case manager compared with those assigned to a regular case manager. Burns and her colleagues (in press) found that service use was affected by the model of case management employed; however, no difference in symptom reduction was noted. These two studies offer some indication that the type of model used can affect service use and clinical outcomes.

In the two studies by Evans and her colleagues, system issues were examined. The first of these studies (Evans, Banks, et al., 1994) offers evidence that case management services can increase the time children can be maintained in community settings as opposed to residential settings. In the second study (Evans, Armstrong, et al., 1994), there are indications that children receiving intensive case management services at home with their families achieved outcomes similar to those of children placed in a therapeutic foster care program.

Clearly, research on case management services research is in its infancy. The results of these studies indicate that future researchers in this area need to clearly describe the organizational structure and clinical implementation of the type of case management under investigation. In addition, the resources contained within the system of care in which case management services function also need to be fully described. Both the level of integration within systems and the amount of resources will have a bearing on the effectiveness of case management services.

In discussing the role of case management/service coordination, Illback and Neill (1995) conclude that "service coordination is both vital and viable" (p. 26) within a system of care. The studies presented in this section illustrate the varied functions, models, and target populations that are feasible for case management services. While the initial results may support the viability of their services, the question of whether such services awaits further examination. Studies of implementation integrity as well as on outcomes of clearly specific models of case management services should be the next steps in this research area.

Future Research Efforts

Research in the area of case management services for children is crucial because it is needed to pave the way for current and future policy decisions. Burns et al. (1995) outline a number of relevant issues that can guide future research in the area of case management services for children, including those related to case management, the primary and additional functions of the case manager, appropriate models of case management, the organizational context of case management for children, implementation practices (e.g., caseload size, intensity and duration of services), qualifications of case managers (e.g., levels, skills), and financing. Furthermore, Burns et al. propose that these issues be investigated by employing the evaluation paradigm of structure, process, and outcome. The latter of the three, outcome, is the method used to investigate the effectiveness of case management interventions at both the client and system levels and describes the level of research reviewed throughout this book (Burns et al., 1995). Later stages of research could examine such areas as cost-effectiveness and the effects of various models of case management for specific populations of children and youth.

Burchard and Clarke (1990) have suggested a number of ways in which future research can investigate the effectiveness of individualized care services. First, single-subject designs, in which children act as their own controls, can be utilized to examine the effectiveness of individualized care. Second, studies can incorporate an experimental group design that compares the outcomes for children who have been randomly assigned to either individualized care or component care. Last, children in a community that provides individualized care can be compared with a matched group of children in a community in which individualized care is not available.

REFERENCES

Achenbach, T.M. (1991a). *Manual for the child behavior checklist/4–8 and 1991 profile.* Burlington: University of Vermont, Department of Psychiatry.

Achenbach, T.M. (1991b). *Manual for the Youth Self-Report and 1991 profile.* Burlington: University of Vermont, Department of Psychiatry.

Achenbach, T.M., & Edelbrock, C. (1983). *Manual for the child behavior checklist and revised child behavior profile.* Burlington: University of Vermont, Department of Psychiatry.

Achenbach, T.M., & Edelbrock, C. (1986). *Manual for the teacher's report form and teacher version of the child behavior profile.* Burlington: University of Vermont, Department of Psychiatry.

American Psychiatric Association. (1987). *Diagnostic and statistical manual of mental disorders* (3rd ed., rev.). Washington, DC: Author.

Angold, A., Cox, A., Prendergast, M., Rutter, M., & Simonoff, E. (1992). *The Child and Adolescent Psychiatric Assessment (CAPA).* Durham, NC: Duke University Medical Center.

Angold, A., Stangl, D., Burns, B.J., Costello, E.J., Tweed, D., & Messer, S.C. (1995). *Perceived family burden resulting from childhood and adolescent psychiatric disorders.* Manuscript submitted for publication.

Austin, C. (1983). Case management in long-term care: Options and opportunities. *Health and Social Work, 8*(1), 16–30.

Behar, L. (1985). Changing patterns of state responsibility: A case study of North Carolina. *Journal of Clinical Child Psychology, 14,* 188–195.

Bigelow, D.A., & Young, D.J. (1991). Effectiveness of a case management program. *Community Mental Health Journal, 27*(2), 115–123.

Burchard, J.D., Burchard, S.N., Sewell, R., & VanDenBerg, J. (1993, August). *One kid at a time: Evaluative case studies and descriptions of the Alaska Youth Initiative Demonstration Project.* Washington, DC: Georgetown University Press.

Burchard, J.D., & Clarke, R.T. (1990). The role of individualized care in a service delivery system for children and adolescents with severely maladjusted behavior. *Journal of Mental Health Administration, 17*(1), 48–60.

Burns, B.J., Angold, A., Magruder-Habib, K., Costello, E.J., & Patrick, M.K.S. (1992). *The Child and Adolescent Services Assessment (CASA).* Durham, NC: Duke University Medical Center.

Burns, B.J., Farmer, E.M.Z., Angold, A., Costello, E.J., & Behar, L. (in press). A randomized trial of case management for youths with serious emotional disturbances. *Journal of Consulting and Clinical Psychology.*

Burns, B.J., & Friedman, R.M. (1990). Examining the research base for children's mental health services and policy. *Journal of Mental Health Administration, 17*(1), 87–98.

Burns, B.J., Gwaltney, E.A., & Bishop, G.K. (1995). Case management research: Issues and directions. In B.J. Friesen & J. Poertner (Eds.), *From case management to service coordination for children with emotional, behavioral, or mental disorders: Building on family strengths* (pp. 353–372). Baltimore: Paul H. Brookes Publishing Co.

Cauce, A.M., Morgan, C.J., Wagner,V., Moore, E., Sy, J., Wurzbacher, K., Weeden, K., Tomlin, S., & Blanchard, T. (1994). Effectiveness of intensive case management for homeless adolescents: Results of a three month follow-up. *Journal of Emotional and Behavioral Disorders, 2*(4), 219–227.

Chamberlain, R., & Rapp, C.A. (1991). A decade of case management: A methodological review of outcome research. *Community Mental Health Journal, 27*(3), 171–188.

Clark, H.B., Prange, M.E., Lee, B., Boyd, L.A., McDonald, B.A., & Stewart, E.S. (1994). Improving adjustment outcomes for foster children with emotional and behavioral disorders: Early findings from a controlled study on individualized services. *Journal of Emotional and Behavioral Disorders, 2*(4), 207–218.

Clarke, R.T., Schaefer, M., Burchard, J.D., & Welkowitz, J.W. (1992). Wrapping community-based mental health services around children with severe behavioral disorder: An evaluation of Project Wraparound. *Journal of Child and Family Studies, 1*(3), 241–261.

Des Moines (Iowa) Public Schools. (1991, September). *SUCCESS, Program, Planning/Evaluation Report for 1990–91.* East Lansing, MI: National Center for Research on Teacher Learning. (ERIC Document Reproduction Service No. ED 340 804)

Early, T.J., & Poertner, J. (1995). Examining current approaches to case management for families with children who have serious emotional disorders. In B.J. Friesen & J. Poertner (Eds.), *From case management to service coordination for children with emotional, behavioral, or mental disorders: Building on family strengths* (pp. 37–59). Baltimore: Paul H. Brookes Publishing Co.

Evans, M.E., Armstrong, M.I., Dollard, N., Kuppinger, A.D., Huz, S., & Wood, V.M. (1994). Development of an evaluation of treatment foster care and family-centered intensive case management in New York. *Journal of Emotional and Behavioral Disorders, 2*(4), 228–239.

Evans, M.E., Banks, S.M., Huz, S., & McNulty, T.L. (1994). Initial hospitalization and community tenure outcomes of intensive case management for children and youth with serious emotional and behavioral disabilities. *Journal of Child and Family Studies, 3*(2), 225–234.

Evans, M.E., Dollard, N., & McNulty, T.L. (1992). Characteristics of seriously emotionally disturbed youth with and without substance abuse in intensive case management. *Journal of Child and Family Studies, 1*(3), 305–314.

Friesen, B.J., & Poertner, J. (Eds.). (1995). *From case management to service coordination for children with emotional, behavioral, or mental disorders: Building on family strengths.* Baltimore: Paul H. Brookes Publishing Co.

Garland, C., Woodruff, G., & Buck, D.M. (1988). *Case management.* Reston, VA: Division for Early Childhood, Council for Exceptional Children.

Goyette, C.H., Connors, C.K., & Ulrich, R.F. (1978). Normative data on revised Connors parent and teacher rating scales. *Journal of Abnormal Child Psychology, 6*(2), 221–236.

Hodges, K. (1993). *Manual for the Child and Adolescent Functional Assessment Scale.* Unpublished manuscript.

Illback, R.J. & Neill, T.K. (1995). Service coordination in mental health systems for children, youth, and families: Progress, problems, prospects. *Journal of Mental Health Administration, 22*(1), 17–28.

188 / WHAT WORKS IN CHILDREN'S MENTAL HEALTH SERVICES?

Intagliata, J., & Baker, F. (1983). Factors affecting case management services for the chronically mentally ill. *Administration in Mental Health, 11*, 75–91.

Katz-Leavy, J.W., Lourie, I.S., Stroul, B.A., & Zeigler-Dendy, C. (1992). Individualizing services in a system of care. In *Profiles of local systems of care for children and adolescents with serious emotional disorders*. Washington, DC: Georgetown University Child Development Center, National Technical Assistance Center for Children's Mental Health.

Kendall, P.C., & Wilcox, L.E. (1979). Self-control in children: Development of a rating scale. *Journal of Consulting and Clinical Psychology, 47*, 1020–1029.

Magura, S., & Moses, B.S. (1986). *Outcome measures for child welfare services: Theory and applications*. Washington, DC: Child Welfare League of America.

Marcenko, M.O., & Smith, L.K. (1992). The impact of a family-centered case management approach. *Social Work in Health Care, 17*(1), 87–100.

Muller, J.B., Jenkins, W.O., Day, C., Schumacher, J.E., Glass, D., Hamilton, G., Mello, M., & Roberson-Hill, D. (1992). Comparative interventions for high risk youth and their families: Outcome results of the JANUS Demonstration Project. In K. Kutash, C.J. Liberton, A. Algarin, & R.M. Friedman (Eds.), *The 5th Annual Research Conference Proceedings, A System of Care for Children's Mental Health: Expanding the Research Base* (pp. 217–223). Tampa: University of South Florida, Florida Mental Health Institute, Research and Training Center for Children's Mental Health.

Patrick, M., Angold, A., Burns, B.J., & Costello, E.J. (1992). *The Child and Adolescent Burden Assessment*. Durham, NC: Duke University Medical Center.

Paulson, R., Gratton, J., Stuntzer-Gibson, D., & Summers, R. (1995, June). *Oregon Partners Project: Progress and outcomes report*. Paper presented at the Building on Family Strengths Conference, Portland, OR.

Research and Training Center for Children's Mental Health. (1988). Individualizing services. *Update, 3*(2), 10–12.

Robinson, G. (1991). Choices in case management. *Community Support Network News, 7*(3), 1, 11–12.

Robinson G.K., & Toff-Bergman, G. (1989). *Choices in case management: Current knowledge and practice for mental health programs*. Washington, DC: Mental Health Policy Resource Center.

Rosen, L.D., Heckman, T., Carro, M.G., & Burchard, J.D. (1994). Satisfaction, involvement, and unconditional care: The perceptions of children and adolescents receiving wraparound services. *Journal of Child and Family Studies, 3*(1), 55–67.

Rubin, A. (1992). Is case management effective for people with serious mental illness? A research review. *Health and Social Work, 17*(2), 138–150.

Singer, G.H., Irvin, L.K., Irvine, B., Hawkins, N., & Cooley, E. (1989). Evaluation of community-based support services for families of persons with developmental disabilities. *Journal of The Association for Persons with Severe Handicaps, 14*(4), 312–323.

Solomon, P. (1992). The efficacy of case management services for severely mentally disabled clients. *Community Mental Health Journal, 28*(3), 163–180.

Stoep, A.V., & Blanchard, T. (1992). Introduction of mental health case management to homeless youth in King County, Washington. In K. Kutash, C.J. Liberton, A. Algarin, & R.M. Friedman (Eds.), *The 5th Annual Re-*

Summary and Conclusion

Child and adolescent mental health is an often neglected area of research (Kazdin, 1993); however, research in the area of children's mental health services has received increased attention since the 1980s. Since the review by Burns and Friedman (1990), the research base examining the effectiveness of the components within a system of care has expanded considerably. The purpose of this book is to provide an overview of the emerging research base and to serve as a catalyst for future research. The information contained in this series of reviews focused on the following children's mental health service components in a system of care: outpatient (psychotherapy) treatment, day treatment, home-based care, therapeutic foster care, crisis and emergency treatment, and residential services and also the two operational services of family support and case management/service coordination. A summary of the findings for each is presented.

In general, most laboratory-based studies of the effectiveness of outpatient psychotherapy for children found an overall positive effect of treatment. However, it has been argued that these laboratory-based studies fail to accurately represent how therapy and treatment are carried out in "real world" clinic-based settings (Kazdin, Bass, Ayers, & Rodgers, 1990; Weisz, 1988; Weisz, Donenberg, Han, & Kauneckis, 1995). In fact, the clinic-based studies reviewed by Weisz and his colleagues seemed to indicate that the effects of psychotherapy are not as positive as the findings reported by the meta-analyses of laboratory-based studies. Because the clinic-based studies, most of which are dated, represent a small database, definite conclusions about the effectiveness of clinic-based, compared with laboratory-based, therapy cannot yet be drawn. Thus, future research must expand the base of research on clinic-based psychotherapy and identify those conditions under which the positive effects of psychotherapy can best be achieved. Furthermore, a limited number of studies have been conducted to examine the *specific* treatment approaches that result in beneficial effects for *specific* types of problems. Additional research is needed which seeks to determine those therapeutic approaches that work most effectively with specific populations of children.

Because features of day treatment programs vary widely in regard to treatment setting, populations served, treatment approaches, theoretical orientations, and program components, our ability to draw conclusive statements concerning effectiveness is limited. However, three *tentative* conclusions appear to be suggested in the research contained in the present review. First, the family plays a significant role in the child's outcome after completion of day treatment services. That is, the involvement of the family in the treatment of the child has a significant impact on outcome. Second, day treatment services appear to be effective for a limited population of children. Most studies found that treatment gains were less likely for children with serious behavior problems than for those with other disorders. Finally, based on a small number of studies, evidence seemed to suggest that treatment gains apparent in the home did not generalize to the school setting. However, emerging school-based mental health service programs may lead to improved outcomes in school settings. Future research in this area must focus upon determining the characteristics of the children and families that benefit most from this treatment approach, the areas of functioning that are most affected by day treatment services, and the components or features of day treatment that are most effective.

Studies evaluating home-based services show that an estimated 70%–96% of the children remained with their families at service termination. Whereas it appears that many home-based programs have proven effective in keeping families intact and preventing or delaying the placement of children, the effects do not appear to be long-lasting, and families continue to be at-risk following service termination. That is, treatment gains decrease as the amount of time after discharge increases. Although these findings appear to support the efficacy of home-based services, concerns have been raised, including the use of a single-outcome criterion (i.e., rate of placement prevention) and the ambiguity associated with the use of placement as an indicator of treatment failure (Wells & Whittington, 1993). Furthermore, Usher (1993) asserts that imprecise targeting of admissions to family preservation programs and inconsistency in service delivery are problematic issues in the evaluation of effectiveness. These issues must be taken into consideration in future research endeavors.

Therapeutic foster care (TFC) services are a relatively new form of treatment for children with serious emotional disorders and their families. The majority of studies conducted in this area have examined discharge rates as the sole outcome criterion, resulting in rates ranging from 62% to 89%. That is, between 62% and 89% of the children who received therapeutic foster care services were placed in less restrictive settings upon discharge. In addition to discharge rates, a limited number of studies have investigated the effects of therapeutic foster care services on other areas, such as child functioning (Chamberlain & Reid, 1991; Chamberlain & Weinrott, 1990; Jones, 1990; Maryland Department of Human Resources, 1987), time spent in family-based settings (Chamberlain & Reid, 1991; Chamberlain & Weinrott, 1990), and rates of incarceration and arrests (Chamberlain, 1990; Chamberlain & Weinrott, 1990). In general, these studies have reported favorable outcomes for TFC on these dimensions; however, only two conducted by Chamberlain and colleagues utilized controlled designs to examine the effectiveness of TFC in comparison with other forms of treatment. The results from these two studies are mixed; one showed no differences in community tenure at follow-up (Chamberlain & Reid, 1991; Chamberlain & Weinrott, 1990), whereas the other found significantly lower rates of incarceration and length of time incarcerated, during treatment and follow-up, for youth enrolled in TFC programs (Chamberlain, 1990; Chamberlain & Weinrott, 1990). Future research topics include establishing the populations for which this service works best, comparing the effectiveness of TFC across multiple dimensions, determining the variables necessary to produce successful outcomes, and examining long-term effects.

Because of the nature of crisis and emergency services, most programs have not included a formal evaluation component. Thus, few studies or evaluations examining the effectiveness of crisis and emergency services are available. Most evaluations examined out-of-home placement prevention rates or the percentage of reduction in admissions to residential settings as outcome criteria. For studies included in this review, placement prevention rates ranged from 60% to 90%. An extensive study (Gutstein, Rudd, Graham, & Rayha, 1988) that examined individual and family functioning and behavioral indicators revealed that children experienced fewer behavioral problems during treatment and follow-up and that family and marital functioning improved. Future research that evaluates the effectiveness of crisis services across multiple dimensions as well as in comparison with other treatment approaches is needed.

Studies investigating the outcomes and efficacy of residential placement (i.e., psychiatric hospitals and residential treatment centers) vary widely in focus and methodology. The majority have not examined residential care in comparison with other service approaches, but rather are descriptive in nature. Factors found to be predictive of a positive outcome included adequate intelligence; nonpsychotic, nonorganic diagnoses; the absence of bizarre and antisocial behaviors; healthy family functioning; adequate length of stay; adequate aftercare; the presence of a standardized treatment regimen; residing with a family member at admission; and parental involvement during treatment (see Blotcky, Dimperio, & Gossett, 1984; Pfeiffer & Strzelecki, 1990; Parmelee et al. 1995). Hoagwood and Cunningham (1992) found that shorter lengths of stay were associated with positive outcome. Factors found to be predictive of poor outcome included a diagnosis of attention-deficit/hyperactivity disorder (ADHD), poor initial response to treatment, older age at admission, child depression or sadness, presence of neurological or psychotic symptoms, limited aftercare services, history of physical abuse, and higher intellectual functioning (Blumberg, 1992; Kalko, 1992). Studies that compared residential treatment services with no-treatment groups found that, in general, youth receiving residential services experienced more positive outcomes than youth who received no services (see Curry, 1991; Dalton, Muller, & Forman, 1988). A limited number of studies have examined the effectiveness of residential services compared with alternative methods. Currently, no evidence exists to support the effectiveness of residential services over other types (see Burns & Friedman, 1990; Cornsweet, 1990; Curry, 1991). Furthermore, a few studies have compared specific therapeutic approaches and have found mixed results. Additional research is needed to determine which youth can most benefit from this type of treatment as well as those treatment approaches that work best with specific populations of children and youth.

A review of family support services, focused specifically on families of children with emotional and behavioral problems, revealed only two evaluations. The evaluations in this developing area generally revealed positive outcomes for parents (see Agosta, 1992; Friesen & Wahlers, 1993). Parents who received family support services were satisfied overall with services received, experienced a positive impact on various family life domains, reported a significant reduction in stress and in family needs in areas specifically addressed by the program, and indicated an increase in coping skills and the ability to maintain their child in the home. Evaluations of outcomes associated with participation in self-help/support groups for families of children with emotional and behavioral disorders also indicated generally positive results. The results of three studies indicated that a large percentage of parents who participated in a self-help/support group reported emotional support as the most beneficial outcome of their participation (see Friesen, 1990; Koroloff & Friesen, 1991; Sheridan & Moore, 1991).

These survey results correspond with the program evaluation results of the Parents Involved Network (PIN) program (Corp & Kosinski, 1991; Fine & Borden, 1992), which revealed that parent participation in the self-help group met parents' support needs; increased self-esteem; and reduced feelings of isolation, guilt, and anger. Furthermore, the results of these program evaluations found that parents who were frequently in contact with support groups or participated in training activities were able to become more effective advocates and gain desirable services for their children. Additional studies have focused on group models that provide both support *and* education for parents of children with emotional or behavioral disorders. Findings revealed that parents reported a more positive self-perception and an increased ability to understand and interact with their children in a competent manner (Dreier & Lewis, 1991). Only one of these studies (Heflinger, 1995) was conducted using an experimental design. Results revealed that participants in the experimental group increased not only their knowledge of mental health service delivery but also their self-efficacy in dealing with the mental health service delivery system as compared with a control group.

The research contained in this review points to a number of possible directions: 1) increase documentation of the needs of families; 2) develop methods and strategies for increasing family involvement and supporting families in their role as "allies"; 3) ascertain more completely the effects of participation in self-help and support groups for families, parents, and siblings; 4) determine *which* group approaches and models (e.g., psychoeducational, support) work most effectively with *which* families; and 5) begin to involve families in the research planning process.

Case management services, also known as service coordination, are one of the newer and more complex approaches for working with children and families. In two studies, Clark et al. (1994) and Paulson, Gratton, Stuntzer-Gibson, and Summers (1995) compared youth receiving case management services with youth who did not receive such services. Whereas Paulson and his colleagues (1995) found increased service coordination and integration for the case management group, no differences were found between groups on measures of psychopathology. Conversely, Clark et al. (1994) found symptom reduction in a few areas; however, outcomes were not examined in terms of service integration and coordination.

In two other studies on case management services, Burns, Farmer, Angold, Costello, and Behar (in press) and Cauce et al. (1994) examined outcomes associated with different models of case management services. An initial analysis by Cauce and her colleagues found some positive differences in psychological and social adjustment for youth assigned to an intensive case manager compared with youth assigned to a regular case manager. Burns and her colleagues (in press) found that service use was affected by the model of case management employed; however, no difference in symptom reduction was noted. These two studies offer some evidence that the type of case management model used can affect service use and clinical outcomes.

In the two studies of case management services conducted by Evans and her colleagues, system issues were examined. The first of these studies (Evans, Banks, Huz, & McNulty, 1994) offers evidence that case management services can increase the amount of time that children are maintained in community settings as opposed to residential settings. In the second study (Evans, Armstrong, et al., 1994), there were indications that children receiving intensive case management services at home with their families achieved outcomes similar to those of children placed in a TFC program.

Case management services generally have been found to result in positive outcomes for other populations of children (e.g., children with developmental disabilities and ongoing health conditions, homeless children and youth, at-risk children and youth, youth with substance abuse problems).

The closely related area of individualized care also suffers from a lack of efficacy studies. Results have been mixed for programs incorporating the principle of individualized care for children and youth with serious emotional disorders. Evaluations of the Willie M. Program in North Carolina did not provide strong support for the reduction of risk of later arrest among violent and assaultive youth following participation in the program. In contrast, a qualitative analysis of 10 youth who participated in the Alaska Youth Initiative revealed that the provision of individualized care was effective in serving as an alternative to restrictive residential treatment for a sample of the most challenging youth in Alaska.

A number of studies have evaluated the effectiveness of Project Wraparound in Vermont. One study indicated the effectiveness of the program in improving child and family functioning in the home setting; however, behavioral improvements did not generalize to the school setting (Clarke, Schaefer, Burchard, & Welkowitz, 1992). Rosen, Heckman, Carro, and Burchard (1994) examined client satisfaction as an outcome for youth ($N = 20$) who received community-based, wraparound services in Vermont and found that the relationship between satisfaction and behavioral adjustment was equivocal; however, the authors concluded that the youths' perceptions of unconditional care did appear to contribute to behavioral adjustment. Yoe, Bruns, and Burchard (1995) investigated the level of restrictiveness in living arrangements and educational placements for 40 youth upon entry and again 12 months after entry into the program. Overall, at the end of 12 months, youth tended to move to less restrictive living and educational environments, with 90% successfully maintained in the community over the 12-month period. Furthermore, an average cost of $4,036 per month for each child receiving individualized services was found (Tighe & Brooks, 1995).

SERVICE SYSTEM RESEARCH VERSUS RESEARCH ON INDIVIDUAL COMPONENTS

Although the research base for each component and operational service was reviewed and discussed separately, in reality the components are more likely to work in combination. This interaction, if planned, becomes a coordinated, possibly integrated comprehensive system of services. Unlike discrete units of service that lend themselves to commonly used experimental research designs, comprehensive service systems "become a menu of possibilities, accompanied by a series of supports that facilitate consumers' interaction with these possibilities" (Knapp, 1995, p. 7). Along with examining the effectiveness of the service components, it is also necessary to conduct research that focuses on the system of services as a unit of analysis (Burns & Friedman, 1990). Because the components of a system of services are interrelated, the effectiveness of an individual component may differ when placed within a system containing other components. For example, the positive long-term effects of residential services may be increased if day treatment services are available as an aftercare service. Therefore, service components must also be viewed within the context or system of which they are part.

SERVICE SYSTEM RESEARCH

Evaluation and research activities in the children's mental health services have only recently incorporated a systems approach (Morrissey, 1992). As treatment for serious emotional disorders in the 1960s moved to the community, so did evaluation and research activities on service delivery. The historic model that included the examination of unitary dimensions of treatment on specific disorders, such as the effects of social skills training on antisocial personality disorders, is being augmented with complex models of interactions among community, service delivery systems, and the family. However, service delivery systems research has received limited attention from researchers in operationalizing and measuring effectiveness and functioning and therefore has lagged behind research on individual service components (Burns, 1994).

There are four salient domains that set or underscore the context for systems of care research:

• Service delivery as movement through an individualized array of services
• Involvement of all child-serving agencies and systems
• Focus on functional impairment as well as diagnosis
• Community characteristics and beliefs

As previously mentioned, an important context for systems of care research is the movement of children and families through a complex array of individualized services usually provided by multiple agencies. This movement may differ for each child and family depending upon individual needs. This movement is illustrated in a recent examination of services and supports received by youth with emotional and behavioral disorders ($n = 134$) who were served in five intensive, community-based programs (see Duchnowski, Johnson, Hall, Kutash, & Friedman, 1993, for a description of the Alternatives to Residential Treatment Study). Using a grid containing 66 discrete service units, parents or caregivers for each youth were asked about use of services during the first 12 months of the program. On average, the number of different service units used was 14, with a range of 5–29 services (Duchnowski, Hall, Kutash, & Friedman, 1995). Services ranged from involvement in Big Brothers/Big Sisters to admission to hospitals and residential treatment centers. Furthermore, 50% of the parents or caregivers indicated that between 14 and 29 service units were received per youth during this 12-month period. This single investigation lends insight into the enormous array of services and supports that can be utilized when supporting youth with emotional and behavioral disorders and their families. Because of the increased complexity in service delivery, evaluation and research efforts also are increasing in complexity.

This service complexity requires the involvement of all child-serving agencies and systems. This context suggests going beyond the mental health service delivery system and integrating other systems, such as juvenile justice, child welfare, education, and public health, into service delivery and research designs. This approach would necessitate extending beyond measures of emotional and behavioral adjustment or symptom reduction to include multiple areas of functioning, including educational and social areas. This approach also implies obtaining multiple perspectives from service providers, parents, teachers, and the children themselves about services and their effects.

A broadly defined target population is the next context for system of care research. The federal definition for children with a "serious emotional disturbance," published by the Substance Abuse and Mental Health Services Administration, Center for Mental Health Services (1993), is as follows:

> persons from birth up to age 18 who currently or at any time during the last year have had a diagnosable mental, behavioral, or emotional disorder of sufficient duration to meet diagnostic criteria specified within DSM-III-R (or the most recent edition of DSM) that resulted in functional impairment which substantially interferes with or limits the child's role or functioning in family, school, or community activities. (p. 29425)

This definition of serious emotional disturbance incorporates the need to examine functional impairment along with diagnostic criteria in estimating prevalence and identification rates. This broad-based definition of impairment has been difficult to operationalize, and the development of instruments to measure impairment is in its infancy. In a survey of 44 state directors of children's mental health programs, 22 directors (50%) reported the inconsistent use of impairment measures on a statewide basis to assist in estimating the prevalence of youth with serious emotional disturbances in their state (Hodges & Gust, 1995).

The final context for systems of care research is the community in which services are delivered. Community descriptions should go beyond the geographic and demographic descriptions that are commonly used and take into account the strengths, problems, natural supports, values, norms, and social and political structures within a community. For example, communities may differ in values and help-seeking behaviors. Such differences can affect a community's responsiveness to interventions and, thus, the manner in which interventions should be structured.

Burns (1994) has suggested that three levels within the framework that have driven the assessment of quality of care at the client level may be adapted and applied to systems research. The first two levels are the structure (organization and linkages between child-serving agencies) and the process (e.g., timeliness of care, appropriateness of care) within systems of care. The third level is outcomes at both the client and system levels, which have received the majority of attention in systems of care research. Three general outcome domains or dependent variables that are examined in systems of care research are described below:

- *Access and utilization of services:* Many studies focus on this single domain of describing the children and youth who use specific services. However, the prevalence of serious emotional disorders in youth is much greater than the utilization of services. Additionally, some services are used more than others, and there is differential use of services (e.g., underutilization of mental health services by African Americans). Access and utilization of services at the system level is a research area needing attention.
- *Costs associated with care:* Another important variable in systems of care research is the cost of service delivery. Other topics within this dependent variable are costs as-

sociated with nonservice or no treatment, costs of multiple service use, and cost shifting from one area to another.

- *Effectiveness or outcomes:* The most popular and most often examined area is the overall effectiveness or outcomes of systems of care. This type of research examines service impact on children and families and systemic outcomes, such as the number of children in out-of-home care before and after the implementation of systems of care. An example of the systemic outcomes or goals of the current systems reform efforts in California has been simplified in the phrase "at home, in school and out-of-trouble" (Rosenblatt, 1993, p. 275). Other areas to explore are satisfaction with services by family members and the children themselves and the often overlooked area of the satisfaction of service providers within systems of care.

To date, only a handful of studies exist that incorporate a systems approach in research on children's mental health (see Stroul, 1993, for a review of these studies). Currently, four efforts in this area employ a control group. These include the California AB377 replication research on the Ventura Model (Rosenblatt, Attkinson, & Fernandez, 1992), Tennessee's Assessment and Intake Management Systems (AIMS) Project (Glisson, 1993; Glisson & James, 1992), the West Virginia Mountain State Network Project (Rugs, Warner-Levock, Johnston, & Freedman, 1994), and the Ft. Bragg Child and Adolescent Mental Health Demonstration Project (Bickman et al., 1995).

The results from the work being conducted in California, Tennessee, and West Virginia suggest that implementation of nontraditional services, especially intensive case management, home-based services, and therapeutic foster care, is effective in altering service-level outcomes. These service-level outcomes include reductions in the number of changes in residential placements experienced by youth, reducing out-of-home care or placement avoidance, and shifting the intensity of treatment from hospitals to communities. However, in studies of service effectiveness, positive clinical outcomes have been harder to obtain. Only the Ft. Bragg project has implemented all three outcome domains of utilization of services, costs, and overall effectiveness. The results of the Ft. Bragg evaluation are mixed; see Friedman and Burns (1996) for a discussion of these results.

FUTURE RESEARCH EFFORTS

Research in the area of children's mental health services is in its infancy; however, the research base is beginning to expand. One important part of this expanding research base has been the examination of the effectiveness of the components within a system of care (Burns, 1994; Burns & Friedman, 1990). It also is necessary to conduct effectiveness research that focuses on the system of care as a unit of analysis (Burns & Friedman, 1990).

Specific research directions for each of the service components discussed in this book are noted at the end of each chapter; however, there are several general research directions that extend the research on the effectiveness of components within a system of care and on the effectiveness of systems of care. It should be acknowledged that the outcomes within systems of care research are dependent upon the outcomes of the individual components that comprise the systems of care. Systems efforts are aimed at reducing out-of-home placements, for example; but individual components operating within the system must demonstrate clinical effectiveness, or the system outcomes are meaningless. Therefore, simultaneous efforts must be made to document the clinical and functional outcomes associated with individual components (and the interaction between them) as well as to show how these efforts contribute to the overall effectiveness of the system of care (see Table 1).

This mutual dependency between component and system outcomes will continue to be a challenge to researchers. Often the role of the researcher is not one of objective isolation but rather of intensive involvement in service system development. Therefore, researchers are responsible for helping to document the goals and delivery of services as well as their outcomes. In order to accomplish this, researchers need to 1) document the "theory of action" (Patton, 1978) or "program theory" (Bickman, 1987) that is occurring within and

Table 1. Goals and outcomes for individual components and systems of care and the shared goals

Individual components	Both components and systems	Systems of care
Clinical improvement	Coordination and integration of services	Access and utilization of services
Improved functioning	Satisfaction with services	Improved functioning
Well-being of child and family and quality of life	Appropriate care	Appropriate use of out-of-home care
Safety of family and child	Quality care	Safety of community
Cost of service	Family involvement	Cost of care

among the interventions so that researchers, participants, and providers understand or agree upon the underlying logic of the intervention; and 2) document and describe the interventions operating in sufficient detail to allow replication of the intervention, including the theoretical underpinning of the employed techniques as well as the intensity of the intervention.

Other research areas and topics abound within children's mental health services. One fertile area is the development of research studies surrounding the topic of cultural competence and the delivery of services that are culturally sensitive. Effectiveness research efforts should begin to include measures of the degree to which services are delivered in a culturally competent manner.

Another future research arena concerns the need to reach beyond systems of care and examine the impact on community outcomes. The examination of multiple outcome criteria, such as children's social and emotional functioning as well as the number of different living arrangements experienced by the child, have begun to be included in studies of the effectiveness of systems of care; however, future investigators may want to include community outcomes in their investigations. For example, evaluations of systems of care could be expanded to include outcome indicators such as decreased school dropout rates within the community, a decreased number of children placed in detention centers, decreased overall rates of child abuse and neglect, and greater involvement of children and families in community activities. The examination of different organizations of systems of care for different types of community configurations is another potential research direction. Systems of care models should be adapted or developed to meet the unique needs of communities. Just as the individual needs of a child and family should be met within a system of care, so should the unique needs of a community.

A need also exists to go beyond having consumers and parents participate in service delivery and research only through the completion of questionnaires dealing with global perceptions of satisfaction with services after services are delivered. Methods of participatory research for parents and consumers should be developed to ensure that they are an integral part of the service delivery, the development of systems of care, the development of research design, and the implementation of the design.

IMPLICATIONS FOR SERVICE DELIVERY

This book began with a summary of two distinct levels at which effectiveness of systems of care can be investigated. The first level entails the more traditional program evaluation strategies of examining and describing the feasibility, acceptability, and general usefulness of an intervention. One of the striking findings from the review of the studies of nontraditional services, especially intensive case management, home-based services, and therapeutic foster care, is that children with severe emotional disorders can be cared for within the community in homelike settings. Beginning in 1985 with efforts surrounding the Willie M. Program (Behar, 1985), programs have demonstrated and continue to demonstrate that the intensity of services, once thought only to exist in hospital or residential care settings, can be delivered in community-based settings.

Furthermore, this intensity of service has been applied to children and adolescents who have emotional and behavioral disturbances that severely limit their functioning in community life. In a field as new as mental health services for children, the accomplishment of successfully serving children and youth with serious emotional disturbances in the community should be acknowledged. When the array of studies in the nontraditional components is examined, the studies clearly document that these components are serving the intended audience of children and youth with severe emotional disturbances and their families. Therefore, service providers and service delivery planners should acknowledge the advancement of the service delivery system in serving children and youth with serious emotional disturbances in community-based settings.

Another implication for the service delivery system is that, although the majority of studies reviewed in this book are not highly controlled experiments, many of the components do point to success for some children and families. Whereas researchers will continue to work with practitioners and family members on documenting what works for whom, at the program level, there is sufficient evidence to support the continued investigation of the broader, systemic issues associated with community-based care for children. This finding is coupled with the overall impression from the studies reviewed that there is no quick fix to helping children with serious emotional disorders and their families. Finally, the results of the reviewed studies are encouraging given that the principles of community-based care for children are relatively new. These principles, established in the early 1980s, have just begun to be operationalized and clearly have some research results that should encourage policy makers and practitioners to further the development of these service mechanisms and to continue to investigate their effectiveness.

CONCLUSIONS

In a 1995 article by Hoagwood, Hibbs, Brent, and Jensen, the authors remind us that knowledge development is not a linear or accretionary process, as has been the case in the development of effective service delivery systems for children with serious emotional disorders. They quote Ernest Cassirer (1955), who warned many years ago:

> The road does not lead solely from "data" to "laws" and from laws back to "axioms" and "principles": the axioms and principles themselves, which at a certain stage of knowledge represent the

ultimate and most complete solution, must once more become a problem. (p. 74)

As the services research base continues to expand, so do the challenges inherent in conducting research on child and adolescent mental health services. However, it is only through the examination of what we do know that we can begin to understand what we do not know. This review has attempted to provide an overview of what we do know and, based on this knowledge, to provide possible avenues for future research endeavors.

REFERENCES

Agosta, J. (1992). Building a comprehensive support system for families. In A. Algarin & R.M. Friedman (Eds.), *The 4th Annual Research Conference Proceedings, A System of Care for Children's Mental Health: Expanding the Research Base* (pp. 3–16). Tampa: University of South Florida, Florida Mental Health Institute, Research and Training Center for Children's Mental Health.

Behar, L. (1985). Changing patterns of state responsibility: A case study of North Carolina. *Journal of Clinical Child Psychology, 14,* 188–195.

Bickman, L. (Ed.). (1987). *Using program theory in evaluation.* San Francisco: Jossey-Bass.

Bickman, L., Guthrie, P.R., Foster, E.M., Lambert, E.W., Summerfelt, W.T., Breda, C.S., & Heflinger, C.A. (1995). *Evaluating managed mental health services: The Ft. Bragg Experiment.* New York: Plenum.

Blotcky, M.J., Dimperio, T.L., & Gossett, J.T. (1984). Follow-up of children treated in psychiatric hospitals: A review of studies. *American Journal of Psychiatry, 141,* 1499–1507.

Blumberg, S. (1992). Initial behavior problems as predictors of outcome in a children's psychiatric hospital. In A. Algarin & R.M. Friedman (Eds.), *The 4th Annual Research Conference Proceedings, A System of Care for Children's Mental Health: Expanding the Research Base* (pp. 185–188). Tampa: University of South Florida, Florida Mental Health Institute, Research and Training Center for Children's Mental Health.

Burns, B.J. (1994). The challenges of child mental health services research. *Journal of Emotional and Behavioral Disorders, 2*(4), 254–259.

Burns, B.J., Farmer, E.M.Z., Angold, A., Costello, E.J., & Behar, L. (in press). A randomized trial of case management for youths with serious emotional disturbances. *Journal of Consulting and Clinical Psychology.*

Burns, B.J., & Friedman, R.M. (1990). Examining the research base for children's mental health services and policy. *Journal of Mental Health Administration, 17*(1), 87–98.

Cassirer, E. (1955). *The philosophy of symbolic forms: Vol. I. Language.* New Haven, CT: Yale University Press.

Cauce, A.M., Morgan, C.J., Wagner, V., Moore, E., Sy, J., Wurzbacher, K., Weeden, K., Tomlin, S., & Blanchard, T. (1994). Effectiveness of intensive case management for homeless adolescents: Results of a three month follow-up. *Journal of Emotional and Behavioral Disorders, 2*(4), 219–227.

Chamberlain, P. (1990). Comparative evaluation of specialized foster care for seriously delinquent youths: A first step. *Community Alternatives: International Journal of Family Care, 2*(2), 21–36.

Chamberlain, P., & Reid, J.B. (1991). Using a specialized foster care community treatment model for children and adolescents leaving the state mental hospital. *Journal of Community Psychology, 19*(3), 266–276.

Chamberlain, P., & Weinrott, M. (1990). Specialized foster care: Treating seriously emotionally disturbed children. *Children Today, 19*(1), 24–27.

Clark, H.B., Prange, M.E., Lee, B., Boyd, L.A., McDonald, B.A., & Stewart, E.S. (1994). Improving adjustment outcomes for foster children with emotional and behavioral disorders: Early findings from a controlled study on individualized services. *Journal of Emotional and Behavioral Disorders, 2*(4), 207–218.

Clarke, R.T., Schaefer, M., Burchard, J.D., & Welkowitz, J.W. (1992). Wrapping community-based mental health services around children with severe behavioral disorder: An evaluation of Project Wraparound. *Journal of Child and Family Studies, 1*(3), 241–261.

Cornsweet, C. (1990). A review of research on hospital treatment of children and adolescents. *Bulletin of the Menninger Clinic, 54*(1), 64–77.

Corp, C., & Kosinski, P. (1991). Parents Involved Network, Delaware County, Pennsylvania Chapter: A self-help, advocacy, information and training resource for parents of children with serious emotional problems. In A. Algarin & R.M. Friedman (Eds.), *The 3rd Annual Research Conference Proceedings, A System of Care for Children's Mental Health: Building a Research Base* (pp. 241–247). Tampa: University of South Florida, Florida Mental Health Institute, Research and Training Center for Children's Mental Health.

Curry, J.F. (1991). Outcome research on residential treatment: Implications and suggested directions. *American Journal of Orthopsychiatry, 61*(3), 348–357.

Dalton, R., Muller, B., & Forman, M. (1988). The psychiatric hospitalization of children: An overview. *Child Psychiatry and Human Development, 19*(4), 231–244.

Dreier, M.P., & Lewis, M.G. (1991). Support and psychoeducation for parents of hospitalized mentally ill children. *Health and Social Work, 16*(1), 11–18.

Duchnowski, A.J., Hall, K.S., Kutash, K., & Friedman, R.M. (1995). *The alternatives to residential treatment study.* Manuscript submitted for review.

Duchnowski, A.J., Johnson, M.K., Hall, K.S., Kutash, K., & Friedman, R.M. (1993). The Alternatives to residential treatment study: Initial findings. *Journal of Emotional and Behavioral Disorders, 1*(1), 17–26.

Evans, M.E., Armstrong, M.I., Dollard, N., Kuppinger, A.D., Huz, S., & Wood, V.M. (1994). Development of an evaluation of treatment foster care and family-centered intensive case management in New York. *Journal of Emotional and Behavioral Disorders, 2*(4), 228–239.

Evans, M.E., Banks, S.M., Huz, S., & McNulty, T.L. (1994). Initial hospitalization and community tenure outcomes of intensive case management for children and youth with serious emotional and behavioral disabilities. *Journal of Child and Family Studies, 3*(2), 225–234.

Fine, G., & Borden, J.R. (1992). Parents Involved Network Project (PIN): Outcomes of parent involvement in support group and advocacy activities. In A. Algarin & R.M. Friedman (Eds.), *The 4th Annual Research Con-*

ference Proceedings, A System of Care for Children's Mental Health: Expanding the Research Base (pp. 25–29). Tampa: University of South Florida, Florida Mental Health Institute, Research and Training Center for Children's Mental Health.

Friedman, R.M., & Burns, B.J. (1996). The evaluation of the Ft. Bragg Demonstration Project: An alternative interpretation of the findings. Journal of Mental Health Administration, 23(1), 128–136.

Friesen, B.J. (1990). National study of parents whose children have serious emotional disorders: Preliminary findings. In A. Algarin, R. Friedman, A. Duchnowski, K. Kutash, S. Silver, & M. Johnson (Eds.), Second Annual Conference Proceedings on Children's Mental Health Services and Policy: Building a Research Base (pp. 29–44). Tampa: University of South Florida, Florida Mental Health Institute, Research and Training Center for Children's Mental Health.

Friesen, B.J., & Wahlers, D. (1993). Respect and real help: Family support and children's mental health. Journal of Emotional and Behavioral Problems, 2(4), 12–15.

Glisson, C. (1993). The adjudication, placement and psychosocial functioning of children in state custody. Unpublished manuscript.

Glisson, C., & James, L. (1992). The interorganizational coordination of services to children in state custody. Administration in Social Work, 3/4, 65–80.

Gutstein, S.E., Rudd, M.D., Graham, J.C., & Rayha, L.L. (1988). Systemic crisis intervention as a response to adolescent crises: An outcome study. Family Process, 27(2), 201–211.

Heflinger, C.A. (1995). Studying family empowerment and parental involvement in their child's mental health treatment. Focal Point, 9(1), 6–8.

Hoagwood, K., & Cunningham, M. (1992). Outcomes of children with emotional disturbance in residential treatment for educational purposes. Journal of Child and Family Studies, 1(2), 129–140.

Hoagwood, K., Hibbs, E., Brent, D., & Jensen, P. (1995). Introduction to the special section: Efficacy and effectiveness in studies of child and adolescent psychotherapy. Journal of Consulting and Clinical Psychology, 63(5), 683–687.

Hodges, K., & Gust, J. (1995). Measures of impairment for children and adolescents. Journal of Mental Health Administration, 22(4), 403–413.

Jones, R.J. (1990). Evaluating therapeutic foster care. In P. Meadowcroft & B.A. Trout (Eds.), Troubled youth in treatment homes: A handbook of therapeutic foster care (pp. 143–181). Washington, DC: Child Welfare League of America.

Kalko, D.J. (1992). Short-term follow-up of child psychiatric hospitalization: Clinical description, predictors, and correlates. Journal of the American Academy of Child and Adolescent Psychiatry, 31(4), 719–727.

Kazdin, A.E. (1993). Adolescent mental health: Prevention and treatment programs. American Psychologist, 48(2), 127–141.

Kazdin, A.E., Bass, D., Ayers, W.A., & Rodgers, A. (1990). Empirical and clinical focus of child and adolescent psychotherapy research. Journal of Consulting and Clinical Psychology, 58, 729–740.

Knapp, M.S. (1995). How shall we study comprehensive services for children and families? Educational Researcher, 24(4), 5–16.

Koroloff, N.M., & Friesen, B.J. (1991). Support groups for parents of children with emotional disorders: A comparison of members and nonmembers. Community Mental Health Journal, 27(4), 265–279.

Maryland Department of Human Resources. (1987). *Specialized foster care.* Baltimore: Department of Fiscal Services.

Morrissey, J.P. (1992). An interorganizational network approach to evaluating children's mental health service systems. In L. Bickman & D. Rog (Eds.), *Evaluating mental health services for children* (pp. 85–98). San Francisco: Jossey-Bass.

Parmelee, D.X., Cohen, R., Nemil, M., Best, A.M., Cassell, S., & Dyson, F. (1995). Children and adolescents discharged from public psychiatric hospitals: Evaluation of outcome in a continuum of care. *Journal of Child and Family Studies, 4*(1), 43–55.

Patton, M.Q. (1978). *Utilization-focused evaluation.* Beverly Hills, CA: Sage Publications.

Paulson, R., Gratton, J., Stuntzer-Gibson, D., & Summers, R. (1995, June). *Oregon Partners Project: Progress and outcomes report.* Paper presented at the Building on Family Strengths Conference, Portland, OR.

Pfeiffer, S.I., & Strzelecki, S. (1990). Inpatient psychiatric treatment of children and adolescents: A review of outcome studies. *Journal of the American Academy of Child and Adolescent Psychiatry, 29*(6), 847–853.

Rosen, L.D., Heckman, T., Carro, M.G., & Burchard, J.D. (1994). Satisfaction, involvement, and unconditional care: The perceptions of children and adolescents receiving wraparound services. *Journal of Child and Family Studies, 3*(1), 55–67.

Rosenblatt, A. (1993). In home, in school, and out of trouble. *Journal of Child and Family Studies, 2*(14), 275–282.

Rosenblatt, A., Attkinson, C.C., & Fernandez, A.J. (1992). Integrating systems of care in California for youth with severe emotional disturbance. II: Initial group home expenditure and utilization findings from the California AB377 evaluation project. *Journal of Child and Family Studies, 1*(3), 263–286.

Rugs, D., Warner-Levock, V., Johnston, A., & Freedman, G. (1994). *Adding system supports to children's service delivery: The impact on foster care children in rural West Virginia.* Unpublished manuscript.

Sheridan, A., & Moore, L.M. (1991). Running groups for parents with schizophrenic adolescents: Initial experiences and plans for the future. *Journal of Adolescence, 14,* 1–16.

Stroul, B.A. (1993). *Systems of care for children and adolescents with severe emotional disturbances: What are the results?* Washington, DC: Georgetown University Child Development Center, National Technical Assistance Center for Children's Mental Health.

Substance Abuse and Mental Health Services Administration, Center for Mental Health Services. (1993, May). In *Federal Register* (pp. 29244–29425). Washington, DC: U.S. Department of Health & Human Services, Office of Human Development.

Tighe, T.A., & Brooks, T. (1995). Evaluating individualized services in Vermont: Intensity and patterns of services, costs, and financing. In C.J. Liberton, K. Kutash, & R.M. Friedman (Eds.), *The 7th Annual Research Conference Proceedings, A System of Care for Children's Mental Health: Expanding the Research Base* (pp. 47–52). Tampa: University of South Florida, Florida Mental Health Institute, Research and Training Center for Children's Mental Health.

Usher, L. (1993, October). *Balancing stakeholder interests in evaluations of innovative programs to serve families and children.* Paper presented at the annual meeting of the Association for Policy Analysis and Management, Washington, DC.

Weisz, J.R. (1988). Assessing outcomes of child mental health services. *Conference Proceedings on Children's Mental Health Services and Policy: Building a Research Base* (pp. 38–43). Tampa: University of South Florida, Florida Mental Health Institute, Research and Training Center for Children's Mental Health.

Weisz, J.R., Donenberg, G.R., Han, S.S., & Kauneckis, D. (1995). Child and adolescent psychotherapy outcomes in experiments versus clinics: Why the disparity? *Journal of Abnormal Child Psychology, 23*(1), 83–106.

Wells, K., & Whittington, D. (1993). Child and family functioning after intensive family preservation services. *Social Service Review, 67*(1), 55–83.

Yoe, J.T., Bruns, E., & Burchard, J. (1995). Evaluating individualized services in Vermont: Behavioral and service outcomes. In C.J. Liberton, K. Kutash, & R.M. Friedman (Eds.), *The 7th Annual Research Conference Proceedings, A System of Care for Children's Mental Health: Expanding the Research Base* (pp. 9–14). Tampa: University of South Florida, Florida Mental Health Institute, Research and Training Center for Children's Mental Health.

Author Index

Page numbers followed by "n" indicate footnotes.

Subject Index

Page numbers followed by "f" or "t" indicate figures or tables, respectively.